Birthmarks of Medical Significance

Guest Editors

BETH A. DROLET, MD
MARIA C. GARZON, MD

PEDIATRIC CLINICS
OF NORTH AMERICA

www.pediatric.theclinics.com

October 2010 • Volume 57 • Number 5

SAUNDERS an imprint of ELSEVIER, Inc.

W.B. SAUNDERS COMPANY
A Division of Elsevier Inc.

1600 John F. Kennedy Boulevard • Suite 1800 • Philadelphia, Pennsylvania 19103-2899

http://www.theclinics.com

THE PEDIATRIC CLINICS OF NORTH AMERICA Volume 57, Number 5
October 2010 ISSN 0031-3955, ISBN-13: 978-1-4377-1854-6

Editor: Carla Holloway

The Pediatric Clinics of North America (ISSN 0031-3955) is published bimonthly by Elsevier Inc., 360 Park Avenue South, New York, NY 10010-1710. Months of issue are February, April, June, August, October, and December. Periodicals postage paid at New York, NY and additional mailing offices. Subscription prices are $167.00 per year (US individuals), $378.00 per year (US institutions), $227.00 per year (Canadian individuals), $503.00 per year (Canadian institutions), $270.00 per year (international individuals), $503.00 per year (international institutions), $83.00 per year (US students and residents), and $142.00 per year (international and Canadian residents and students). To receive students/resident rare, orders must be accompanied by name of affiliated institution, date of term, and the signature of program/residency coordinator on institution letterhead. Orders will be billed at individual rate until proof of status is received. Foreign air speed delivery is included in all *Clinics* subscription prices. All prices are subject to change without notice. **POSTMASTER:** Send address changes to *The Pediatric Clinics of North America*, Elsevier Health Sciences Division, Subscription Customer Service, 3251 Riverport Lane, Maryland Heights, MO 63043. **Customer Service: 1-800-654-2452 (US and Canada). From outside of the US and Canada: 1-314-447-8871. Fax: 1-314-447-8029. For print support, E-mail: JournalsCustomerService-usa@elsevier.com. For online support, E-mail: JournalsOnlineSupport-usa@elsevier.com.**

Reprints. For copies of 100 or more, of articles in this publication, please contact the Commercial Reprints Department, Elsevier Inc., 360 Park Avenue South, New York, NY 10010-1710. Tel.: 212-633-3812; Fax: 212-462-1935; E-mail: reprints@elsevier.com.

The Pediatric Clinics of North America is also published in Spanish by McGraw-Hill Inter-americana Editores S.A., Mexico City, Mexico; in Portuguese by Riechmann and Affonso Editores, Rua Comandante Coelho 1085, CEP 21250, Rio de Janeiro, Brazil; and in Greek by Althayia SA, Athens, Greece.

The Pediatric Clinics of North America is covered in *MEDLINE/PubMed (Index Medicus), Excerpta Medica, Current Contents; Current Contents/Clinical Medicine, Science Citation Index, ASCA, ISI/BIOMED*, and *BIOSIS*.

Printed and bound in the United Kingdom

Transferred to Digital Print 2011

GOAL STATEMENT

The goal of *Pediatric Clinics of North America* is to keep practicing physicians up to date with current clinical practice in pediatrics by providing timely articles reviewing the state of the art in patient care.

ACCREDITATION

The *Pediatric Clinics of North America* is planned and implemented in accordance with the Essential Areas and Policies of the Accreditation Council for Continuing Medical Education (ACCME) through the joint sponsorship of the University Of Virginia School Of Medicine and Elsevier. The University Of Virginia School of Medicine is accredited by the ACCME to provide continuing medical education for physicians.

The University of Virginia School of Medicine designates this educational activity for a maximum of 15 *AMA PRA Category 1 Credits*™ for each issue, 90 credits per year. Physicians should only claim credit commensurate with the extent of their participation in the activity.

The American Medical Association has determined that physicians not licensed in the US who participate in this CME activity are eligible for a maximum of 15 *AMA PRA Category 1 Credits*™ for each issue, 90 credits per year.

Credit can be earned by reading the text material, taking the CME examination online at http://www.theclinics.com/home/cme, and completing the evaluation. After taking the test, you will be required to review any and all incorrect answers. Following completion of the test and evaluation, your credit will be awarded and you may print your certificate.

FACULTY DISCLOSURE/CONFLICT OF INTEREST

The University of Virginia School of Medicine, as an ACCME accredited provider, endorses and strives to comply with the Accreditation Council for Continuing Medical Education (ACCME) Standards of Commercial Support, Commonwealth of Virginia statutes, University of Virginia policies and procedures, and associated federal and private regulations and guidelines on the need for disclosure and monitoring of proprietary and financial interests that may affect the scientific integrity and balance of content delivered in continuing medical education activities under our auspices.

The University of Virginia School of Medicine requires that all CME activities accredited through this institution be developed independently and be scientifically rigorous, balanced and objective in the presentation/discussion of its content, theories and practices.

All authors/editors participating in an accredited CME activity are expected to disclose to the readers relevant financial relationships with commercial entities occurring within the past 12 months (such as grants or research support, employee, consultant, stock holder, member of speakers bureau, etc.). The University of Virginia School of Medicine will employ appropriate mechanisms to resolve potential conflicts of interest to maintain the standards of fair and balanced education to the reader. Questions about specific strategies can be directed to the Office of Continuing Medical Education, University of Virginia School of Medicine, Charlottesville, Virginia.

The faculty and staff of the University of Virginia Office of Continuing Medical Education have no financial affiliations to disclose.

The authors/editors listed below have identified no financial or professional relationships for themselves or their spouse/partner:

Heather A. Brandling-Bennett, MD; Beth A. Drolet, MD (Guest Editor); Kelly Duffy, PhD; Carla Holloway, (Acquisitions Editor); Jennifer T. Huang, MD; Michael Kelly, MD, PhD; Valerie B. Lyon, MD; Karen Rheuban, MD (Test Author); Kara N. Shah, MD, PhD; and James Treat, MD.

The authors/editors listed below identified the following professional or financial affiliations for themselves or their spouse/partner:

Maria Garzon, MD (Guest Editor) is an industry funded research/investigator for Astellas and RegeneRX.
Kristen E. Holland, MD's spouse is employed by Abbott Laboratories.
Marilyn G. Liang, MD is an industry funded research/investigator for Pierre Fabre Dermatologie.
Kimberly D. Morel, MD is an industry funded research/investigator for Astellas and RegeneRX.

Disclosure of Discussion of Non-FDA Approved Uses for Pharmaceutical Products and/or Medical Devices
The University of Virginia School of Medicine, as an ACCME provider, requires that all faculty presenters identify and disclose any off-label uses for pharmaceutical and medical device products. The University of Virginia School of Medicine recommends that each physician fully review all the available data on new products or procedures prior to clinical use.

TO ENROLL

To enroll in the Pediatric Clinics of North America Continuing Medical Education program, call customer service at 1-800-654-2452 or visit us online at http://www.theclinics.com/home/cme. The CME program is available to subscribers for an additional fee of $223.00.

Contributors

GUEST EDITORS

BETH A. DROLET, MD
Professor and Vice Chairman of Dermatology; Professor of Pediatrics, Medical College of Wisconsin; Medical Director of Dermatology and Birthmarks and Vascular Anomalies, Children's Hospital of Wisconsin, Milwaukee, Wisconsin

MARIA C. GARZON, MD
Professor of Clinical Dermatology and Clinical Pediatrics Columbia University; Director, Pediatric Dermatology Morgan Stanley Children's Hospital, New York Presbyterian, New York, New York

AUTHORS

HEATHER A. BRANDLING-BENNETT, MD
Assistant Professor, University of Washington; Attending Dermatologist, Seattle Children's Hospital, Seattle, Washington

BETH A. DROLET, MD
Professor and Vice Chairman of Dermatology; Professor of Pediatrics, Medical College of Wisconsin; Medical Director of Dermatology and Birthmarks and Vascular Anomalies, Children's Hospital of Wisconsin, Milwaukee, Wisconsin

KELLY DUFFY, PhD
Assistant Professor, Dermatology Department, Pediatric Dermatology, Medical College of Wisconsin, Milwaukee, Wisconsin

KRISTEN E. HOLLAND, MD
Assistant Professor, Department of Dermatology, Medical College of Wisconsin; Children's Hospital of Wisconsin, Milwaukee, Wisconsin

JENNIFER T. HUANG, MD
Department of Dermatology, Harvard Medical School; Clinical Fellow in Pediatric Dermatology, Dermatology Program, Children's Hospital Boston, Boston, Massachusetts

MICHAEL KELLY, MD, PhD
Associate Professor of Pediatrics, Department of Pediatrics, Division of Hematology/Oncology/Bone Marrow Transplant, Medical College of Wisconsin; Cancer Program Director, Children's Hospital of Wisconsin, Milwaukee, Wisconsin

MARILYN G. LIANG, MD
Assistant Professor, Department of Dermatology, Harvard Medical School; Dermatology Program, Children's Hospital Boston, Boston, Massachusetts

VALERIE B. LYON, MD
Assistant Professor of Dermatology and Pediatrics; Director, Pediatric Dermatologic
Surgery and Skin Oncology, Department of Dermatology, Medical College of Wisconsin,
Children's Hospital of Wisconsin, Milwaukee, Wisconsin

KIMBERLY D. MOREL, MD
Assistant Professor of Clinical Dermatology and Clinical Pediatrics, Department
of Dermatology, Morgan Stanley Children's Hospital of New York Presbyterian,
Columbia University, New York, New York

KARA N. SHAH, MD, PhD
Assistant Professor of Pediatrics and Dermatology, University of Pennsylvania
School of Medicine; Attending Physician, Section of Pediatric Dermatology,
Division of General Pediatrics, The Children's Hospital of Philadelphia,
Philadelphia, Pennsylvania

JAMES TREAT, MD
Assistant Professor of Pediatrics and Dermatology, Department of Pediatrics,
Section of Dermatology, University of Pennsylvania School of Medicine, Children's
Hospital of Philadelphia, Philadelphia, Pennsylvania

Contents

Infantile hemangiomas (IHs) are the most common soft tissue tumors of childhood. The wide spectrum of disease has made it difficult to predict need for treatment and has made it challenging to establish a standardized approach to management. This article provides the reader with an up-to-date discussion of IH, identifying features of this condition which predict need for treatment as well as associated complications and reviewing management.

The objective of this article is to provide a comprehensive overview of the Kasabach-Merritt Phenomenon. The clinical presentation, laboratory findings, vascular pathology, and pathophysiology are discussed.

Vascular malformations are rare but important skin disorders in children, which often require multidisciplinary care. The goal of this article is to orient pediatricians to the various types of vascular malformations. We discuss the clinical characteristics, diagnostic criteria, and management of capillary, venous, arteriovenous, and lymphatic malformations. Associated findings and syndromes are also discussed briefly.

Historically, vascular malformations were not thought to be the result of genetic abnormalities because most of those presenting clinically are sporadic. However, research in this field has expanded over the last decade, leading to the identification of genetic defects responsible for several inherited forms of vascular malformations and associated syndromes, which has shed light on the pathogenesis of sporadic lesions. This advancement in the field has not only enhanced diagnostic capabilities but also improved our understanding of the potential role of complex genetic mechanisms in vascular malformation development. This article focuses on genetic contributions of vascular malformations in the context of syndromes and the tests that are available.

The terms *pigmentary mosaicism* or *patterned dyspigmentation* describe a spectrum of clinical findings that range from localized areas of dyspigmentation with no systemic findings to widespread dyspigmentation with associated neurologic, musculoskeletal, and cardiac abnormalities, and other sequelae that can lead to early demise. Given this wide spectrum, these patients must be approached with caution, but with the understanding that most who have localized pigmentary anomalies, such as segmental pigmentary disorder (SegPD) seem to have no systemic manifestations. These patients can be approached in many different ways, but generally children with more widespread dyspigmentation, and any with associated abnormalities or not meeting neurodevelopmental milestones, should be evaluated closely. Children with any red flags warrant subspecialty referral, and all children deserve close clinical follow-up with their primary care physician to ensure they meet all of their developmental milestones. Fortunately, parents can be reassured that most children with SegPD, and many with more widespread patterned pigmentation, are otherwise healthy.

Café-au-lait, also referred to as café-au-lait spots or café-au-lait macules, present as well-circumscribed, evenly pigmented macules and patches that range in size from 1 to 2 mm to greater than 20 cm in greatest diameter. Café-au-lait are common in children. Although most café-au-lait present as 1 or 2 spots in an otherwise healthy child, the presence of multiple café-au-lait, large segmental café-au-lait, associated facial dysmorphism, other cutaneous anomalies, or unusual findings on physical examination should suggest the possibility of an associated syndrome. While neurofibromatosis type 1 is the most common syndrome seen in children with multiple café-au-lait, other syndromes associated with one or more café-au-lait include McCune-Albright syndrome, Legius syndrome, Noonan syndrome and other neuro-cardio-facialcutaneous syndromes, ring chromosome syndromes, and constitutional mismatch repair deficiency syndrome.

The relative risk for melanoma arising within a congenital nevus is related to the size of the lesion. The timing of and clinical presentation of development of melanoma is also related to the size of the lesion. Medical decisions are individualized taking into account the perceived risk of malignancy, psychosocial impact, and anticipated treatment outcome. In this article, the common features of congenital nevi are discussed as well as the potential individual variations and their impact on treatment recommendations.

Epidermal Nevi

Epidermal Nevi

Heather A. Brandling-Bennett and Kimberly D. Morel

> Nevi or nests of cells may be made up of a variety of cell types. The cell types that live in the epidermis include epidermal cells or keratinocytes, sebaceous glands, hair follicles, apocrine and eccrine glands, and smooth muscle cells. This article discusses epidermal or keratinocyte nevi, nevus sebaceous, nevus comedonicus, smooth muscle hamartomas, and inflammatory linear verrucous epidermal nevi. Syndromes associated with epidermal nevi are also reviewed.

THE CLINICS ARE NOW AVAILABLE ONLINE!

Access your subscription at:
www.theclinics.com

Preface

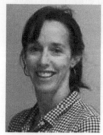 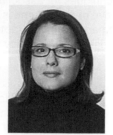

Beth A. Drolet, MD   Maria C. Garzon, MD
Guest Editors

Birthmarks are among the most common types of anomalies encountered by the pediatrician in practice. Moreover, they are a source of significant concern for parents regardless of whether they are associated with an underlying systemic abnormality. Pediatricians are often called upon in the neonatal period to establish the diagnosis and direct management. Recognition of the types of birthmarks that require additional evaluation or herald a potentially problematic course is essential when examining an infant. Once an initial diagnosis is established, the pediatrician's role is to identify the lesions that require additional evaluation or referral to subspecialists, monitor the behavior of the birthmark, and periodically reassess whether the initial diagnosis is the correct one. In order to do this well, it is essential for the physician to recognize that birthmarks represent a heterogeneous group of disorders. Pigmented and vascular birthmarks are very common. Vascular birthmarks occur in many infants with the common fading type vascular stain (nevus simplex salmon patches) being noted in almost half of all newborns. Although less common than nevus simplex, infantile hemangiomas also occur frequently and are encountered routinely in a pediatric practice. In the past, many different types of vascular birthmarks with different biologic behaviors and clinical characteristics have traditionally been grouped together because of similarities in their appearance and the presence of vascular tissue within histologic specimens. The lumping together of vascular disorders (often using the term "hemangioma" to describe them all) with very different biologic behaviors and prognoses hampered our understanding of these diseases and by extension their treatment for decades. Unfortunately the misuse of terminology persists and continues to be the cause of confusion and anxiety for parents of children with vascular birthmarks. By recognizing these potential pitfalls, the evaluating physician can steer families towards the appropriate evaluation. Within the spectrum of pigmented birthmarks there is often great anxiety regarding the potential for malignant transformation or the risk for neurocutaneous disease when an infant has café au lait macules or patterned pigmentation. These concerns can be addressed and in some cases dispelled if an accurate diagnosis is established early in life.

Pediatr Clin N Am 57 (2010) xi–xii
doi:10.1016/j.pcl.2010.08.004
0031-3955/10/$ — see front matter © 2010 Elsevier Inc. All rights reserved.

Over the last decade there has been an explosion in knowledge in the field of birth-marks with an emphasis on clinical features that will predict systemic involvement. In addition, radiologic imaging and screening techniques for associated anomalies have evolved over the last several years. The objective of this volume is to provide pediatri-cians with a comprehensive review of birthmarks with the potential for systemic involvement and birthmarks with increased risk of malignancy and to help guide them in their evaluation and management.

Beth A. Drolet, MD
Children's Hospital of Wisconsin
Department of Dermatology
9000 W. Wisconsin Avenue
Milwaukee, WI 53226, USA

Maria C. Garzon, MD
Columbia University Pediatric Dermatology
161 Fort Washington Avenue
New York, NY 10032, USA

E-mail addresses:
drolet@mcw.edu (B.A. Drolet)
mcg2@columbia.edu (M.C. Garzon)

Infantile Hemangioma

Kristen E. Holland, MD[a],*, Beth A. Drolet, MD[b]

KEYWORDS

- Infantile hemangioma • Treatment • Complications

Infantile hemangiomas (IHs), also known as hemangiomas of infancy, are the most common soft tissue tumors of childhood. Despite their frequency, much remains to be learned about the pathogenesis, and management often is based on anecdote rather than evidence-based data. While most IHs are uncomplicated and do not require intervention, they can be a significant source of parental distress, cosmetic disfigurement, and morbidity. The wide spectrum of disease, both in the morphology of these lesions, but more importantly in their behavior, has made it difficult to predict need for treatment and has made it challenging to establish a standardized approach to management.

The nomenclature surrounding hemangiomas is confusing, as several entities recognized today as distinct vascular tumors or malformations historically have been referred to as hemangiomas. This article focuses on IH, which must be differentiated from congenital hemangioma. Unlike IHs, congenital hemangiomas are well formed at birth, tend to be bulky tumors, and do not undergo proliferation. Similar to IH, a halo of pallor may be present surrounding the lesion, and central ulceration may occur. Some of these lesions undergo rapid involution within the first several months of life (rapidly involuting congenital hemangiomas or RICH), whereas others remain unchanged (noninvoluting congenital hemangiomas or NICH). As congenital hemangiomas are well developed by birth, they may be detected in utero by prenatal ultrasound. Immunohistochemical markers also help distinguish congenital hemangiomas from IH, as they do not stain with GLUT-1.

EPIDEMIOLOGY

There have been few prospective studies performed assessing the exact incidence of IHs. Incidence has been difficult to ascertain, because IHs may not appear until after the immediate newborn period. In addition, the confusing nomenclature and often

[a] Department of Dermatology, Children's Hospital of Wisconsin, Medical College of Wisconsin, Suite B260, 9000 West Wisconsin Avenue, Milwaukee, WI 53226, USA
[b] Children's Hospital of Wisconsin, 9000 West Wisconsin Avenue, Milwaukee, WI 53226, USA
* Corresponding author. Department of Dermatology, Children's Hospital of Wisconsin, Medical College of Wisconsin, Suite B260, 9000 West Wisconsin Avenue, Milwaukee, WI 53226.
E-mail address: kholland@mcw.edu

Pediatr Clin N Am 57 (2010) 1069–1083
doi:10.1016/j.pcl.2010.07.008
0031-3955/10/$ – see front matter © 2010 Elsevier Inc. All rights reserved.

pediatric.theclinics.com

misuse of the term hemangioma make interpretation of older studies difficult. The incidence of IH has been estimated to be 1% to 5%.[1] Risk factors for development of IH include Caucasian ethnicity, low birth weight, and female sex (female to male ratio of 2.4:1).[2,3] Infants who are products of a multiple gestation pregnancy have a higher risk of developing a hemangioma. The incidence of multiple gestation in a large hemangioma population was three times greater compared with that of the general population reported by the National Center for Health Statistics; this finding may be confounded by low birth weight, which is an established independent risk factor.[2,3] IHs previously were considered sporadic; however, clinicians have noted a familial tendency, often caring for multiple siblings with hemangiomas. A recent study observed that 32% of patients with IH had a vascular anomaly in a first-degree relative; familial IH was specifically reported in 12% of patients.[2] Walter and colleagues[4] studied five families (22 individuals) with hemangiomas and vascular malformations and found a linkage to a locus on chromosome 5q31-33. This suggests that genes are located on this part of the chromosome, which contributes to the development of hemangiomas. While these data provide compelling evidence that genetic factors contribute significantly to the development of hemangiomas, to the authors' knowledge, none of these studies have led to identification of a specific gene.

PATHOGENESIS

The pathogenesis of infantile hemangiomas is poorly understood, but is generally believed to be multifactorial. Many studies have analyzed hemangioma tissue from surgical specimens. North and colleagues[5] were first to note that the endothelial-like cells of the hemangioma expressed GLUT-1, the erythrocyte-type glucose transporter protein. This appears to be an exclusive marker for IH and is an invaluable tool used to distinguish hemangiomas from other vascular lesions. GLUT-1 is also expressed on the chorionic villus cells of the placenta, and several studies have pointed out the molecular similarities between placenta and IH. A relationship to the placenta as the possible source of hemangioma endothelial cells also has been suggested given the presence of overlapping markers in both hemangioma and placental vessels.[6]

The rapid proliferation of endothelial-like cells has led many investigators to focus on angiogenesis, in which new vessels develop from local endothelial cells. Alternatively, there is evidence that IHs may develop through vasculogenesis, in which new vessels arise from circulating endothelial progenitor cells recruited to hypoxic tissue.[7] Children with proliferating IHs have increased levels of circulating endothelial progenitor cells and surgical specimens of hemangiomas are positive for the coexpression of progenitor specific markers such as CD34, CD133, and vascular endothelial growth factor (VEGF) receptor-2.[7–9]

Molecular and cellular mediators have been implicated in the proliferative and involutive phases of hemangiomas VEGF, basic fibroblast growth factor, insulin-like growth factor-2, tissue inhibitor of metalloproteinase (TIMP) type 1, type 4 collagenase, urokinase, hypoxia-inducible growth factor (HIF1alpha), and mast cells.[5,8] It recently was noted that the VEGF signaling pathway may play an important role in the development of IHs. Recent studies suggest that a shift in the balance of VEGF to VEGF receptor binding results in endothelial proliferation within IHs.[10]

CLINICAL

IHs have tremendous clinical heterogeneity in their appearance and behavior. These lesions vary in presentation from small, red lesions to large and bulky tumors that place individuals at risk for functional impairment or permanent disfigurement.

Although IHs are considered to be birthmarks, they are often not recognized until a few weeks of age. Unlike traditional birthmarks whose appearance remains relatively stable throughout life, IH demonstrate change over the first months of life. Early on, they can appear as a telangiectatic patch or an area of pallor (**Fig. 1**). Historically, IHs have been classified by their depth of soft tissue involvement (superficial, deep, and mixed).[11–13] Superficial hemangiomas involve the superficial dermis and appear as bright red lesions (**Fig. 2**). These lesions may be plaque-like or more rounded papules or nodules. Deep hemangiomas involve the deep dermis and subcutis, and present as bluish to skin-colored nodules (**Fig. 3**). Mixed hemangiomas have both superficial and deep components, and therefore have features of both (**Fig. 4**). However, another classification based on morphology has proven to be more predictive of risk of complications or need for treatment. Under this classification system, hemangiomas have been described as localized or segmental or indeterminate.[12,13] Localized hemangiomas are discrete and usually oval or round, whereas the term segmental has been used to describe hemangiomas that demonstrate a geographic shape and involve a broad anatomic region or a recognized developmental unit (**Fig. 5**). As segmental hemangiomas are at higher risk of complications and associated anomalies, the distinction is an important one. The concept of a segmental distribution may not be readily familiar to some physicians; however, these lesions can be recognized by their larger size as they have been shown to cover four times greater surface area than localized lesions.[13]

The natural history of IH is characterized by an initial proliferative or growth phase followed by a plateau phase, and finally the involution phase. However, the transition from the growth phase to involution may be more dynamic than previously thought, reflecting a balance between local proliferative factors and factors involved in apoptosis.[14] Most hemangioma growth occurs in the first 5 months, at which point 80% of the final size has often been reached.[14] However, some IHs exhibit minimal proliferation, remain flat, and may be reticular or network-like in appearance. On

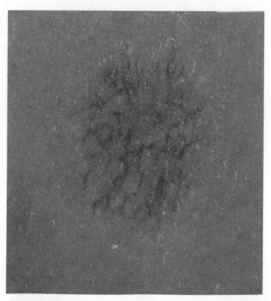

Fig. 1. Early hemangioma in a newborn.

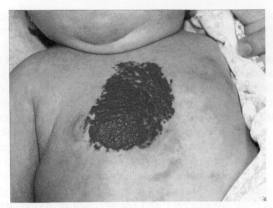

Fig. 2. Superficial hemangioma.

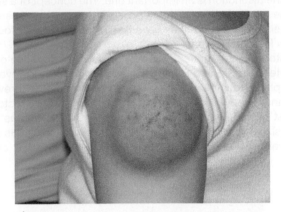

Fig. 3. Deep hemangioma.

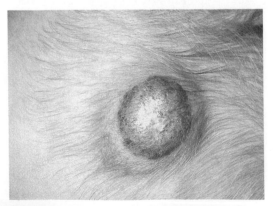

Fig. 4. Mixed hemangioma.

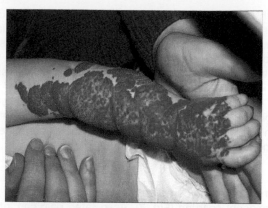

Fig. 5. Segmental hemangioma.

average, IHs typically reach their maximum size by 9 months, but deep hemangiomas may proliferate longer. Prolonged growth for 2 years has been rarely observed. Hemangiomas with an extended growth phase tend to be larger lesions and more often segmental or indeterminate rather than localized.[15] A subset of hemangiomas (23 IHs) evaluated from a large prospective study of 1530 IHs that demonstrated prolonged growth were all of the deep or combined subtype, and it was the deep component that was subjectively felt to have the continued growth in most.[15] In the proliferative phase, IHs tend to be firm and noncompressible, becoming softer and more compressible as they begin to involute (**Fig. 6**). A change in color from bright red to purple or gray can often signal transition to the involution phase. Involution takes place over several years.

IHs may occur anywhere on the skin, but are most common on the head and neck. Reproducible patterns of segmental hemangiomas on the face have been demonstrated and mapped.[12,16] Segmental involvement of the lower face corresponds to known embryologic facial prominences (maxillary, mandibular, and frontonasal), whereas involvement of the upper face (forehead) does not.

COMPLICATIONS

Although most IHs are uncomplicated and do not require treatment, 24% of those referred to tertiary institutions had complications.[17] Providers should be aware of risk factors predictive of complications or need for treatment to facilitate early referral

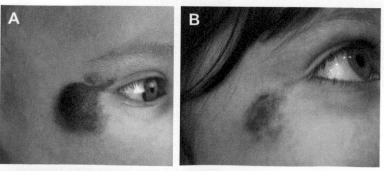

Fig. 6. Hemangioma in proliferative phase (*A*) and involution phase (*B*).

to a physician with expertise in the management of IH. Size, location, and subtype (localized vs segmental) are major factors to consider in evaluating an infant's risk.[17] Specifically, for every 10 cm^2 increase in size, a 5% increase in likelihood of complications and a 4% increase in likelihood of treatment have been reported.[17] Although segmental hemangiomas tend to be larger lesions, this subtype has been shown to be an independent risk factor for the development of complications.[17] Complications of IH include ulceration, functional impairment (visual compromise, airway obstruction, auditory canal obstruction, feeding difficulty), and cardiac compromise. High-risk locations for specific complications, permanent disfigurement, and associated anomalies are outlined in **Table 1**.[14]

Ulceration

Ulceration is the most common complication (16%), and can result in pain, infection, bleeding, and permanent scarring (**Fig. 7**). Associated pain can interfere with sleep and feeding. Locations at high risk for ulceration and the associated frequency of this complication include anogenital (50%), lower lip (30%), and neck (25%).[18] IHs that are larger in size or of the segmental subtype are more likely to develop ulceration. Of the clinical subtypes (ie, superficial, mixed, and deep), the mixed subtype (having both superficial and deep components) has most frequently been associated with ulceration and is another independent risk factor.[18,19] The cause of ulceration is not well understood, but maceration and friction are likely contributing factors given the higher frequency in locations prone to this. While ulceration can be complicated by bleeding, clinically significant bleeding (ie, requiring hospitalization/transfusion) is rare.[18]

Visual Compromise

Complications of periorbital hemangiomas include visual axis obstruction, refractive error (astigmatism or myopia), retrobulbar involvement, amblyopia, and tear duct obstruction. Lesions that involve the posterior orbit result in proptosis or displacement of the globe. Given the threat of permanent visual impairment, patients with periorbital hemangiomas should be referred early to a physician with expertise in the treatment of IH and should be closely monitored by the ophthalmology department; monitoring should include a retinal examination.[20]

Table 1	
Locations at risk for complications from infantile hemangioma	
Location	**Associated Risk**
Periorbital and retrobulbar	Visual axis occlusion, astigmatism, amblyopia
Nasal tip, ear, large facial	Cosmetic disfigurement, scarring
Perioral, lip	Ulceration, feeding difficulties, cosmetic disfigurement
Perineal, axilla, neck	Ulceration
Beard distribution, central neck	Airway hemangioma
Liver, large	High-output heart failure
Large facial ("segmental")	PHACE syndrome (see text)
Multiple hemangiomas	Visceral involvement (liver, gastrointestinal tract most common)
Midline lumbosacral	Tethered spinal cord, intraspinal hemangioma, intraspinal lipoma, genitourinary anomalies

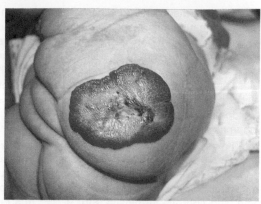

Fig. 7. Ulcerated hemangioma in the diaper region.

Visceral Involvement and Complications

While solitary lesions are most common, multiple cutaneous hemangiomas may occur in 30% of patients, although only 3% of patients have greater than six.[17] Historically patients with numerous lesions have been placed into at least two categories: disseminated neonatal hemangiomatosis and benign neonatal hemangiomatosis, with the former considered to be at the severe end of the spectrum, with multiple sites of potential extracutaneous disease and a mortality rate as high as 60%.[21] However, in the past, all multifocal vascular lesions were considered to be hemangiomas, and with advances in histopathologic and radiologic diagnosis (ie, GLUT-1 stain), it is recognized that some of these severe cases represent other multifocal vascular anomalies rather than true IH. Many of these other multifocal vascular lesions have a more aggressive course, often with coagulopathy and bleeding, and account for the high mortality historically reported with disseminated neonatal hemangiomatosis. In some cases, this has led to overly aggressive intervention in infants with asymptomatic multifocal IH.

Patients with true multifocal cutaneous IH are recognized to have a higher risk of visceral hemangiomas, with liver and gastrointestinal (GI) involvement being most common. Ultrasound of the liver has been recommended in those patients with greater than five cutaneous hemangiomas.[22] A recent prospective study investigated the incidence of hepatic involvement in patients with more than five cutaneous IHs compared with those with one to four cutaneous lesions, and demonstrated a significantly increased risk in patients with greater than five cutaneous lesions. In this study, 24 (16%) of the infants with five or more cutaneous IHs had hepatic hemangiomas, whereas none of the infants with less than five had hepatic hemangiomas ($P<.003$), substantiating the recommendation for liver ultrasound in patients with greater than five cutaneous IHs.[23] Reported complications of liver hemangiomas include high-output heart failure if there is significant arteriovenous shunting (typically large liver lesions), abdominal compartment syndrome, and hypothyroidism. It should be noted that isolated liver involvement without skin lesions also can occur.

Associated Anomalies

The presence of IH in particular locations can be a marker for underlying or associated anomalies. The beard distribution of an IH in which preauricular areas, chin, anterior neck, and lower lip are involved has been associated with airway hemangiomas

(**Fig. 8**). In two retrospective studies, 29% to 63% of patients with large IHs on the lower lip, chin, neck, and preauricular region (beard) had airway involvement.[24,25] Airway hemangiomas typically present between 6 and 12 weeks of age with biphasic inspiratory and expiratory stridor and retractions.[24,26] Cough may be associated and may mimic croup. Infants with IH in the beard distribution should be monitored closely for respiratory difficulties and referred to an ear, nose, and throat specialist for evaluation. Serial evaluations may be required in young infants, since the skin hemangioma may precede the development of symptomatic airway IH.

Cutaneous hemangiomas in the lumbosacral area also have been reported in association with underlying developmental anomalies. As the skin overlying the lumbosacral region has an intimate developmental relationship with the neural tube, hemangiomas in this location have been recognized as one of the cutaneous markers associated with occult spinal dysraphism including tethered cord, lipomyelomeningocele, intraspinal lipoma, and tight fila terminalia (**Fig. 9**).[27,28] In a prospective cohort study evaluating the risk of spinal anomalies in patients with a midline lumbosacral IH, 51% of the patients evaluated by magnetic resonance imaging (MRI) demonstrated spinal anomalies (intraspinal hemangioma or lipoma, structural malformation of the cord, or tethered cord).[29] Of these, 35% had an isolated IH without other signs of spinal dysraphism. This corresponded to a relative risk of spinal anomalies of 640 (children with IH plus another cutaneous sign of spinal dysraphism) and 438 (children with isolated IH). Given the low sensitivity of ultrasound (50%) demonstrated in the aforementioned study, MRI should be performed in these patients to look for these anomalies to prompt early detection and prevention of neurologic impairment. Additional anomalies reported in association with lumbosacral IH include anorectal, urinary tract, and external genitalia malformations.[27,28] These malformations are typically evident at birth, prompting further evaluation to determine the extent of the associated anomalies; however, it has been suggested that systematic pelviperineal imaging should be performed even in the absence of obvious malformations, as the potential for occult anomalies exists.[27]

Large facial hemangiomas have been described in association with posterior fossa brain malformations, arterial cerebrovascular anomalies, cardiovascular anomalies, eye anomalies, and ventral developmental defects, specifically sternal defects or supraumbilical raphe.[30] Posterior fossa malformations, hemangioma, arterial abnormalities, cardiac defects/aortic coarctation, eye abnormalities (PHACE) syndrome refers to the constellation of findings in this neurocutaneous syndrome; recently, diagnostic criteria have been established to more precisely define this syndrome.[31] Little is known about the pathogenesis, natural history, or long-term outcome of PHACE

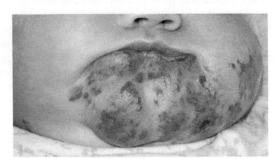

Fig. 8. Hemangioma in a beard distribution with associated underlying airway hemangioma.

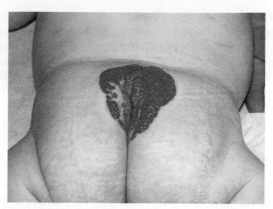

Fig. 9. Lumbosacral hemangioma with underlying tethered cord.

syndrome. There is a strong female predominance, with nearly 90% of cases being female.[32] Unlike isolated IH, patients with PHACE tend to be born full-term, normal birth weight, and singleton, suggesting a different pathogenesis.

Hemangiomas associated with PHACE syndrome tend to be large plaque-like, segmental facial hemangiomas (**Fig. 10**). In a recent prospective study systematically evaluating 108 patients with large facial hemangiomas at risk for PHACE syndrome, 33 (31%) met criteria for PHACE syndrome.[33] Structural cerebral or cerebrovascular anomalies are the most common extracutaneous findings associated with PHACE syndrome, and have been described in 72% of PHACE patients in one study. However, this number may have underestimated the true incidence, as not all at risk patients were thoroughly evaluated for associated anomalies in this study.[32] Using standardized screening with MRI/magnetic resonance angiography (MRA) of the head and neck and echocardiogram, 94% had cerebrovascular anomalies, and 67% had cardiovascular anomalies.[33] Neurologic sequelae including seizures, developmental delay, focal motor impairments, headache, and stroke have been reported.[32] Aortic arch anomalies are the most frequent cardiovascular finding; these anomalies include aortic coarctation, aortic interruption, and tortuous aorta, and are often associated with anomalous subclavian arteries. Ocular and ventral developmental anomalies occur less commonly, reported in 7% to 17% and 5% to 25% of patients,

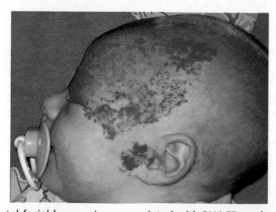

Fig. 10. S1 segmental facial hemangioma associated with PHACE syndrome.

respectively.[32,33] Rarely, endocrine abnormalities may be associated, including structural pituitary anomalies and endocrinopathies including hypopituitarism, hypothyroidism, growth hormone deficiency, and diabetes insipidus.[32] All patients with large facial IH at risk for PHACE syndrome should have thorough investigation of the brain, heart, and eyes to evaluate for PHACE-associated anomalies. Although MRI can demonstrate certain cerebrovascular anomalies, MRA is necessary to fully characterize the cerebrovasculature.

MANAGEMENT

The clinical heterogeneity and unpredictable and variable course of IH complicate management decisions, and have contributed to the lack of an evidenced-based standard of care. There are few prospective studies looking at safety and efficacy of therapies for IH, and no US Food and Drug Administration (FDA)-approved agents for IH exist. As a result, selection of therapeutic modalities is based on anecdote and small case series. Physicians caring for an infant with IH must first determine whether treatment is indicated. Although most hemangiomas are self-limited, up to 38% of hemangiomas referred to tertiary care specialists require systemic treatment due to complications such as ulceration, bleeding, risk for permanent disfigurement, obstruction of vision, airway obstruction, or high-output cardiac failure.[17] Several factors outlined in **Table 2** must be considered by physicians managing patients with IH.

Ulceration

Initial therapy for most ulcerated hemangiomas, common indications for treatment, is local wound care. Gentle debridement of crust overlying the ulceration can be achieved with wet compresses with astringent solutions of aluminum acetate (ie, Domeboro solution [Bayer Health care, Morristown, NJ, USA). In the diaper area, barrier creams containing zinc oxide or petrolatum play an important role in protecting the skin from maceration and irritation from urine and stool, which may inhibit healing. Nonadherent dressings such as petrolatum gauze or extrathin hydrocolloid dressings may act as an additional barrier to outside pathogens or irritants and promote healing. As secondary infection can develop in ulcerated IH, cultures should be obtained in nonhealing lesions, and topical antibiotics (ie, polymyxin-bacitracin, mupirocin, metronidazole) should be employed. Oral antibiotics may be necessary in patients nonresponsive to topical measures.

In ulcerations recalcitrant to initial topical measures outlined previously, topical application of becaplermin gel, a recombinant human platelet-derived growth factor, has been shown in a small case series to be effective at speeding healing.[34] More

Table 2	
Factors to consider in estimating need for treatment	
Therapeutic Consideration	**Intervention More Likely**
Location at risk for complication, functional impairment, cosmetic disfigurement	See **Table 1**
Presence of ulceration	Symptomatic from pain, bleeding
Growth pattern	Rapid or prolonged
Age	Younger age = higher potential for growth Incomplete resolution or presence of residual infantile hemangioma in a school-aged child

recently, a boxed warning was placed on this medication about the possible increased risk of mortality secondary to malignancy in some patients. As a result, its role is generally reserved as a second- or third-line agent for patients who have failed other treatment modalities.

Corticosteroids

Systemic corticosteroids at a dose of 2 to 5 mg/kg/d (typically 2–3 mg/kg/d) historically have been the mainstay of therapy. Response to treatment is variable, with one retrospective study reporting regression in one-third, stabilization of growth in another third, and minimal to no response in the final third.[35] Adverse effects are common, and include irritability, GI upset, sleep disturbance, cushingoid facies, adrenal suppression, immunosuppression, hypertension, bone demineralization, cardiomyopathy, and growth retardation.[36] Catch-up growth occurs in most children once the corticosteroids are discontinued. The duration of treatment and approach to tapering corticosteroids is variable, as it is dependent on the treatment response, age of the child, inherent growth characteristics of the IH, and complications of therapy. For example, younger infants tend to be treated longer (months) given their greater potential for IH growth, whereas older infants whose IH may be nearing the end of its proliferative phase would be less likely to need prolonged therapy. A prospective study of 16 infants evaluating the immunosuppressive effects of corticosteroids demonstrated that both lymphocyte cell numbers and function are affected.[37] As the levels of tetanus and diphtheria antibodies were not found to be protective in 11 and 3 of the patients respectively, it has been recommended that patients who receive oral corticosteroids during the immunization period have these checked and additional immunizations provided if titers are not protective. In addition, prophylaxis with a combination of trimethoprim and sulfamethoxazole should be considered in infants to protect against pneumocystis pneumonia (PCP), as there are reports of PCP in this setting.[38]

Intralesional and topical corticosteroids also have been reported to decrease the size or slow growth of IH.[36] This is most effective for small and localized cutaneous hemangiomas. The efficacy of topical steroids is limited by the depth of their penetration compared with the depth of hemangioma involvement. Doses of intralesional triamcinolone should not exceed 3 to 5 mg/kg per treatment.[36] Repeated injections are often necessary to maintain response. Central retinal artery occlusion, believed to be the result of pressure exceeding systolic pressure during injection, has been reported in the treatment of periocular hemangiomas, limiting triamcinolone's use in this location.[36] Other complications related to intralesional corticosteroids include skin atrophy and necrosis, calcification, and rarely, adrenal suppression (dose-dependent).

Vincristine

Vincristine has been reported to be effective in the treatment of IH, and has historically been reserved for those IH resistant to corticosteroids or in patients intolerant of corticosteroids. Single weekly doses of 1 to 1.5 mg/m^2 resulted in improvement of all nine patients reported by Enjolras.[39–41] Constipation is the most common side effect, but neuromyopathy, most commonly presenting as foot drop, is a potentially serious side effect. Administration of vincristine requires placement of a central line; therefore, risks associated with this must be considered also.

Propranolol

Propranolol has recently been used in the treatment of IHs after growth arrest of an infant's hemangioma was incidentally noted when propranolol was started for obstructive hypertrophic myocardiopathy.[42] Improvement in color, softening, growth arrest, and even regression of IHs have been observed with administration of propranolol.[42,43] Since the initial report, the use of propranolol for IH has soared, as it is perceived to have a lower adverse effect profile than other systemic therapies used for treating IH. Its mechanism of action in the treatment of IH is unknown. Doses of 1 to 3 mg/kg/d divided twice or three times daily are typically used, but clearly outlined and safe protocols for initiation and monitoring do not exist, resulting in a wide range in recommendations. The most common serious adverse effects of propranolol include bradycardia and hypotension. Hypoglycemia, particularly after overnight fast, may be observed.[44] Other adverse effects include bronchospasm (particularly in patients with reactive airway disease), congestive heart failure, depression, nausea, vomiting, abdominal cramping, sleep disturbance, and night terrors.

There are theoretical considerations specific to using oral propranolol for the treatment of IH (Table 3). Regarding hypoglycemia, most patients will be less than 1 year of age, have limited glycogen stores and a relative inability to communicate, recognize, or treat symptoms. Furthermore, low birth weight, an important risk factor for the development of IH, also confers a greater risk of hypoglycemia. Oral corticosteroids are used frequently for the treatment of IHs; during treatment, there may be some protective effect as steroids inhibit insulin action. However, after prolonged steroid use, there may be residual adrenal suppression and subsequent loss of the counter-regulatory cortisol response, thus increasing risk of hypoglycemia. In patients with PHACE syndrome and cerebrovascular or aortic arch anomalies, lower blood pressure may decrease blood flow through stenotic or dysplastic vessels resulting in hypoperfusion of the brain (when cerebrovascular vessels are involved) or the lower body (when aortic coarctation is present). Finally, in patients with high-output cardiac failure secondary to a large liver hemangioma, the use of propranolol could result in

Table 3
Patients with theoretical increased risk of adverse effects from propranolol for infantile hemangioma

Population	Side Effect	Reason for Concern
<1 year of age, particularly LBW infants	Hypoglycemia	Limited glycogen stores Inability to communicate symptoms
Patients previously treated with systemic steroids	Hypoglycemia	Muted counter-regulatory cortisol response secondary to adrenal suppression
PHACE syndrome patients with cerebrovascular anomalies	Hypoperfusion of brain	Narrowed, stenotic vessels may require higher blood pressure for perfusion; propranolol associated with decreased cerebral blood flow
PHACE syndrome patients with aortic arch obstruction	Systemic hypoperfusion	Aortic obstruction may require higher blood pressure to maintain perfusion to segments distal to the obstruction
Hemangioma-related high-output cardiac failure (ie, large liver hemangioma)	Decompensation of heart failure	Decreased heart rate/contractility limits cardiac response to high-output demands

Abbreviation: LBW, low-birth weight.

decompensation secondary to drug-induced suppression of heart rate/contractility. Until the safety of propranolol in these patients can be established and these theoretic concerns allayed, caution should be exercised when prescribing propranolol.

Interferon

Recombinant interferon-alfa, an inhibitor of angiogenesis, administered as a subcutaneous injection of 3 million units per square meter per day, also has been used successfully for the treatment of IH.[36] Adverse effects include influenza-like symptoms of fever, irritability, and malaise. Less commonly, transient neutropenia and liver enzyme abnormalities may develop. Spastic diplegia, irreversible in some cases, also has been a reported side effect. The development of spastic diplegia has been observed more frequently in infants treated at an earlier age, the time at which there is often greatest need for treatment. Consequently, its use is not recommended.

Laser

The pulsed dye laser (PDL) has been successfully used for vascular birthmarks, namely capillary malformations or port-wine stains, for years, and its efficacy in this setting is well established. Its use in the treatment of proliferating IH remains controversial, as adverse outcomes including ulceration and scarring have been described.[45] In addition, the use of PDL for intact IH is limited by the depth of the laser's penetration (1 mm). There are a number of reports and two prospective studies describing its benefit in the treatment of ulcerated hemangiomas both in terms of speeding re-epithelialization as well as decreasing pain.[46,47] The mechanism for this is not well understood. Greatest consensus surrounding the use of the PDL for IH is in the treatment of residual telangiectases after involution, for which the PDL is most effective.

Surgery

Surgical excision may be an option for function- or life-threatening hemangiomas when medical therapy fails or is not tolerated, but more commonly its role is for removal of residual fibrofatty tissue or correction of scarring after involution. Surgical correction may be pursued at an earlier age if it is clear that the child will ultimately need a procedure for the residual effects.

REFERENCES

1. Kilcline C, Frieden IJ. Infantile hemangiomas: how common are they? A systematic review of the medical literature. Pediatr Dermatol 2008;25(2):168–73.
2. Hemangioma Investigator Group, Haggstrom AN, Drolet BA, et al. Prospective study of infantile hemangiomas: demographic, prenatal, and perinatal characteristics. J Pediatr 2007;150(3):291–4.
3. Drolet BA, Swanson EA, Frieden IJ, et al. Infantile hemangiomas: an emerging health issue linked to an increased rate of low birth weight infants. J Pediatr 2008;153(5):712, No-715.
4. Walter JW, Blei F, Anderson JL, et al. Genetic mapping of a novel familial form of infantile hemangioma. Am J Med Genet 1999;82(1):77–83.
5. North PE, Waner M, Mizeracki A, et al. GLUT1: a newly discovered immunohistochemical marker for juvenile hemangiomas. Hum Pathol 2000;31(1):11–22.
6. Barnes CM, Huang S, Kaipainen A, et al. Evidence by molecular profiling for a placental origin of infantile hemangioma. Proc Natl Acad Sci U S A 2005; 102(52):19097–102.

7. Kleinman ME, Greives MR, Churgin SS, et al. Hypoxia-induced mediators of stem/progenitor cell trafficking are increased in children with hemangioma. Arterioscler Thromb Vasc Biol 2007;27(12):2664–70.

8. Dadras SS, North PE, Bertoncini J, et al. Infantile hemangiomas are arrested in an early developmental vascular differentiation state. Mod Pathol 2004;17(9): 1068–79.

9. Yu Y, Flint AF, Mulliken JB, et al. Endothelial progenitor cells in infantile hemangioma. Blood 2004;103(4):1373–5.

10. Jinnin M, Medici D, Park L, et al. Suppressed NFAT-dependent VEGFR1 expression and constitutive VEGFR2 signaling in infantile hemangioma. Nat Med 2008; 14(11):1236–46.

11. Drolet BA, Esterly NB, Frieden IJ. Hemangiomas in children. N Engl J Med 1999; 341(3):173–81.

12. Haggstrom AN, Lammer EJ, Schneider RA, et al. Patterns of infantile hemangiomas: new clues to hemangioma pathogenesis and embryonic facial development. Pediatrics 2006;117(3):698–703.

13. Chiller KG, Passaro D, Frieden IJ. Hemangiomas of infancy: clinical characteristics, morphologic subtypes, and their relationship to race, ethnicity, and sex. Arch Dermatol 2002;138(12):1567–76.

14. Chang LC, Haggstrom AN, Drolet BA, et al. Growth characteristics of infantile hemangiomas: implications for management. Pediatrics 2008;122(2): 360–7.

15. Brandling-Bennett HA, Metry DW, Baselga E, et al. Infantile hemangiomas with unusually prolonged growth phase: a case series. Arch Dermatol 2008;144(12): 1632–7.

16. Waner M, North PE, Scherer KA, et al. The nonrandom distribution of facial hemangiomas. Arch Dermatol 2003;139(7):869–75.

17. Haggstrom AN, Drolet BA, Baselga E, et al. Prospective study of infantile hemangiomas: clinical characteristics predicting complications and treatment. Pediatrics 2006;118(3):882–7.

18. Chamlin SL, Haggstrom AN, Drolet BA, et al. Multicenter prospective study of ulcerated hemangiomas. J Pediatr 2007;151(6):684.

19. Shin HT, Orlow SJ, Chang MW. Ulcerated haemangioma of infancy: a retrospective review of 47 patients. Br J Dermatol 2007;156(5):1050–2.

20. Bilyk JR, Adamis AP, Mulliken JB. Treatment options for periorbital hemangioma of infancy. Int Ophthalmol Clin 1992;32(3):95–109.

21. Golitz LE, Rudikoff J, O'Meara OP. Diffuse neonatal hemangiomatosis. Pediatr Dermatol 1986;3(2):145–52.

22. Dickie B, Dasgupta R, Nair R, et al. Spectrum of hepatic hemangiomas: management and outcome. J Pediatr Surg 2009;44(1):125–33.

23. Horii KA, Drolet BA, Frieden IJ, et al. Prospective study of the frequency of hepatic hemangiomas in infants with multiple cutaneous infantile hemangiomas. Pediatrics, in press.

24. Orlow SJ, Isakoff MS, Blei F. Increased risk of symptomatic hemangiomas of the airway in association with cutaneous hemangiomas in a beard distribution. J Pediatr 1997;131(4):643–6.

25. O TM, Alexander RE, Lando T, et al. Segmental hemangiomas of the upper airway. Laryngoscope 2009;119(11):2242–7.

26. Perkins JA, Duke W, Chen E, et al. Emerging concepts in airway infantile hemangioma assessment and management. Otolaryngol Head Neck Surg 2009;141(2): 207–12.

27. Girard C, Bigorre M, Guillot B, et al. PELVIS syndrome. Arch Dermatol 2006; 142(7):884–8.
28. Stockman A, Boralevi F, Taieb A, et al. SACRAL syndrome: spinal dysraphism, anogenital, cutaneous, renal and urologic anomalies, associated with an angioma of lumbosacral localization. Dermatology 2007;214(1):40–5.
29. Drolet BA, Garzon MC, Adams D, et al. A prospective study of spinal anomalies in children with infantile hemangiomas of the lumbosacral skin. J Pediatr, in press.
30. Frieden IJ, Reese V, Cohen D. PHACE syndrome. The association of posterior fossa brain malformations, hemangiomas, arterial anomalies, coarctation of the aorta and cardiac defects, and eye abnormalities. Arch Dermatol 1996;132(3): 307–11.
31. Metry D, Heyer G, Hess C, et al. Consensus statement on diagnostic criteria for PHACE syndrome. Pediatrics 2009;124(5):1447–56.
32. Metry DW, Haggstrom AN, Drolet BA, et al. A prospective study of PHACE syndrome in infantile hemangiomas: demographic features, clinical findings, and complications. Am J Med Genet A 2006;140(9):975–86.
33. Haggstrom AN, Garzon MC, Baselga E, et al. Risk for PHACE syndrome in infants with large facial hemangiomas. Pediatrics 2010;126(2):e418–26.
34. Metz BJ, Rubenstein MC, Levy ML, et al. Response of ulcerated perineal hemangiomas of infancy to becaplermin gel, a recombinant human platelet-derived growth factor. Arch Dermatol 2004;140(7):867–70.
35. Enjolras O, Riche MC, Merland JJ, et al. Management of alarming hemangiomas in infancy: a review of 25 cases. Pediatrics 1990;85(4):491–8.
36. Barrio VR, Drolet BA. Treatment of hemangiomas of infancy. Dermatol Ther 2005; 18(2):151–9.
37. Kelly ME, Juern AM, Grossman WJ, et al. Immunosuppressive effects in infants treated with corticosteroids for infantile hemangiomas. Arch Dermatol 2010; 146(7):767–74.
38. Maronn ML, Corden T, Drolet BA. Pneumocystis carinii pneumonia in infant treated with oral steroids for hemangioma. Arch Dermatol 2007;143(9):1224–5.
39. Enjolras O, Breviere GM, Roger G, et al. Vincristine treatment for function- and life-threatening infantile hemangioma. Arch Pediatr 2004;11:99–107.
40. Fawcett SL, Grant I, Hall PN, et al. Vincristine as a treatment for a large haemangioma threatening vital functions. Br J Plast Surg 2004;57(2):168–71.
41. Boehm DK, Kobrinsky NL. Treatment of cavernous hemangioma with vincristine. Ann Pharmacother 1993;27(7–8):981.
42. Leaute-Labreze C, Dumas de la Roque E, Hubiche T, et al. Propranolol for severe hemangiomas of infancy. N Engl J Med 2008;358(24):2649–51.
43. Sans V, Dumas de la Roque E, Berge J, et al. Propranolol for severe infantile hemangiomas: follow-up report. Pediatrics 2009.
44. Holland KE, Frieden IJ, Frommelt PC, et al. Hypoglycemia in children taking propranolol for the treatment of infantile hemangioma. Arch Dermatol 2010;146 (7):775–8.
45. Witman PM, Wagner AM, Scherer K, et al. Complications following pulsed dye laser treatment of superficial hemangiomas. Lasers Surg Med 2006;38(2): 116–23.
46. Morelli JG, Tan OT, Yohn JJ, et al. Treatment of ulcerated hemangiomas of infancy. Arch Pediatr Adolesc Med 1994;148(10):1104–5.
47. David LR, Malek MM, Argenta LC. Efficacy of pulse dye laser therapy for the treatment of ulcerated haemangiomas: a review of 78 patients. Br J Plast Surg 2003;56(4):317–27.

Kasabach-Merritt Phenomenon

Michael Kelly, MD, PhD[a,b]

KEYWORDS

- Kasabach-Merritt Phenomenon • Coagulopathy
- Thrombocytopenia • Kaposiform Hemangioendothelioma
- Tufted Angioma

OVERVIEW

Kasabach-Merritt Phenomenon (KMP) is a life-threatening, consumptive coagulopathy associated with an underlying vascular tumor.[1] KMP is characterized by severe thrombocytopenia, microangiopathic anemia, hypofibrinogenaemia, and elevated fibrin split products in the presence of a rapidly enlarging tumor.[2] The coagulopathy is likely related to the sequestration of platelets and clotting factors within the vascular lesion resulting in systemic disseminated intravascular coagulation and a high propensity for patients to clot and bleed.[3] Kasabach and Merritt first described this consumptive coagulopathy in a 2-month-old boy with a giant capillary hemangioma and purpura.[1] However, recent studies support an association of KMP with the vascular tumors kaposiform hemangioendothelioma (KHE) and tufted angioma (TA), not infantile hemangioma.[4–6] The clinical presentation and laboratory findings of KMP, as well as the histopathology and treatment of KMP and the underlying vascular tumors are discussed.

CLINICAL PRESENTATION

KMP typically has its onset early in infancy with a median age of onset of 5 weeks.[7] In approximately 50% of cases, KMP was associated with a vascular tumor diagnosed at birth with 90% of published cases diagnosed before 1 year of age.[4–8] Boys and girls were equally affected. KMP was most often associated with a rapidly growing, large (>5 cm) solitary tumor commonly involving extremities, trunk, or face and neck. Most of these tumors involved subcutaneous and deep structures and were locally invasive. Skin over the tumors was most often described as deep red to purple in color with an advancing ecchymotic rim. The tumors were often warm and leathery to palpation[4] with a nodular feel. Widespread cutaneous petechiae were often seen in subjects

---

[a] Department of Pediatrics, Division of Hematology/Oncology/Bone Marrow Transplant, Medical College of Wisconsin, 8701 Watertown Plank Road, MFRC Suite 3018, Milwaukee, WI 53226, USA
[b] Children's Hospital of Wisconsin, Milwaukee, WI, USA
E-mail address: mekelly@mcw.edu

Pediatr Clin N Am 57 (2010) 1085–1089
doi:10.1016/j.pcl.2010.07.006
0031-3955/10/$ – see front matter © 2010 Elsevier Inc. All rights reserved.

pediatric.theclinics.com

with platelet counts less than 10,000. Signs and symptoms of bleeding were seen in more than 50% of children with KMP at presentation in one report.[8] Subjects with retroperitoneal or visceral lesions presented with abdominal distention, signs of organ dysfunction, or high-output heart failure often without cutaneous signs.[4,6,8]

LABORATORY AND RADIOGRAPHIC FINDINGS

All subjects with KMP had profound thrombocytopenia and hypofibrinogenemia with elevated fibrin split products (D-dimers), suggestive of an active consumptive coagulopathy. Platelet counts at the time of diagnosis ranged from 6000 to 98,000 with fibrinogen levels less than 100 mg/dL; whereas, D-dimers were always greater than 1.[4,6,8] Pretreatment prothrombin times (PT) and activated partial thromboplastin time (PTT) were not routinely measured, but ranged from normal[4] to significantly prolonged.[8] In one series, 80% of subjects presented with anemia at diagnosis.[8] Evidence of intravascular hemolysis, including red blood cell fragmentation, elevated LDH, and hyperbilirubinemia, was a common finding.[9,10]

MRI was the most frequently used modality to assess vascular tumors associated with KMP. These tumors were described as diffusely enhancing masses isointense to muscle on T1-weighted and hyperintense on T2-weighted sequences.[4] The tumors involved multiple tissue planes and had poorly defined margins. Cutaneous thickening and fat stranding were common features.[4] Superficial draining vessels were often dilated, but vessels in the tumor were small and infrequent. Signal voids consistent with hemosiderin deposits were often noted on MRI.[4]

VASCULAR PATHOLOGY ASSOCIATED WITH KMP

Seminal studies in the 1990s challenged the long-held belief that KMP was a complication of infantile hemangiomas[4,5,11] and definitely showed the association of KMP with KHE and TA (**Fig. 1**). Of the 40 biopsy samples from 52 subjects in these studies, 35 were diagnosed with KHE; whereas, 5 were called TA. None had histology or clinical features consistent with infantile hemangioma. Since then, biopsies of most lesions associated with KMP have shared the same histopathologic features.[3,6,8,12] Indeed, the original case described by Kasabach and Merritt of a 2-month-old child with a capillary hemangioma with purpura was likely a KHE.[1]

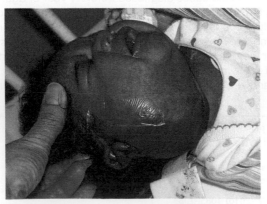

Fig. 1. A 15-day-old girl with large, invasive kaposiform hemangioendothelioma with Kasabach-Merritt syndrome.

KHE is a locally aggressive vascular tumor characterized by sheets and lobules of round and spindle shaped endothelial cells that form crescentic vascular spaces and, less commonly, round capillary-like spaces.[3,11] Superficial tumors infiltrate the dermis and subcutaneous tissues; whereas, deep and visceral lesions extensively involve and entrapp normal adjacent structures. Fibrin and platelet-rich microthrombi are frequently identified within the tumor tissue suggesting areas of platelet trapping and blood destruction.[3] Endothelial cells in the tumor nodules are positive for CD31, CD34, and FLI1, but negative for the hemangioma-specific markers GLUT1 and LeY.[3] TA associated with KMP present as cutaneous lesions with small, discrete nodules of capillary vessels situated in the deep dermis, hypodermis, or both, with an evenly distributed cannonball pattern with peripheral crescentic slitlike vessels and dense fibrosis.[5] Capillary lumens are typically small, lined by attenuated endothelial cells, and often filled with erythrocytes. Both TA and KHE are known to occur in association with lymphatic abnormalities thought to be an intrinsic part of the lesion, not just a result of lymphatic obstruction by the tumor.[3,5,11] The striking similarities in the histologic features of KHE and TA and the observation that both entities have been described within the same tumor[13] have led some to speculate that KHE and TA are the same disease on a continuum.[3–5,13]

Why KMP develops exclusively in the setting of KHE or TA is currently unknown. Lyons and colleagues[3] have speculated that it is the unique architectural or endothelial composition found in KHE and TA that promote platelet trapping and a consumptive coagulopathy. In contrast to the ordered treelike vasculature of infantile hemangioma, convoluted capillaries arise directly off large vessels in KHE and TA resulting in turbulent flow-promoting platelet activation and aggregation. Furthermore, unique characteristics of the endothelial tumor cells within KHE and TA may promote platelet adhesion and activation. However, only a percentage of patients diagnosed with TA or KHE have an associated consumptive coagulopathy, arguing that other features, such as tumor size, may be an important determinant. The observation that most patients diagnosed with KMP are a few weeks or months of age could possibly be explained by proportionately larger tumors in this age group, or suggest other important developmental differences in platelet or endothelial function that may result in an increased susceptibility for development of KMP in young patients with KHE or TA.

TREATMENT

KMP is associated with significant morbidity and mortality. Children with KMP can die of hemorrhage or invasion/compression of vital structures by the tumor. Mortality has ranged between 10% to 30% in most series.[3–6,8,13,14] The management of KMP should include supportive care to maintain hemostasis and curative therapy directed at the treatment of the underlying tumor.

The principle of management of coagulopathy in KMP is to treat patients not numbers.[8] Despite marked thrombocytopenia at presentation, platelet transfusions should be reserved for active bleeding or in preparation for surgery or procedures. Infused platelets have a short circulatory time and have been noted to rapidly increase the size of the tumor and even exacerbate KMP in some cases,[15] presumably through increased platelet trapping within the lesion.[16,17] The use of aminocaproic acid and local measures may be helpful to reduce the need for platelet transfusions in these patients.[18] Antiplatelet agents, such as acetylsalicylic acid and dipyridamole, have been used in an attempt to reduce platelet aggregation within the body of the tumor.[19] Treatment of hypofibrinogenemia with cryoprecipitate and prolonged PT or PTT with fresh frozen plasma should also be a clinical decision rather than correction of a laboratory result.[8] Symptomatic anemia should be treated with red blood cell transfusions.

Successful treatment of the underlying malignancy is critical to the correction of KMP and to the overall survival of patients. Several therapies have been reported for KHE/TA, but none have been uniformly effective. Although surgical removal of the tumor has been associated with immediate normalization of hemostasis and hematologic abnormalities,[20] it is rarely attempted because of the large size and infiltrating nature of KHE/TA associated with KMP. Tumor embolization has been used with some success in combination with medical and surgical therapies.[8] Medical therapies have included corticosteroids, alpha interferon (IFN), vincristine (VCR), and other chemotherapy agents used alone and in combination[21–23] with varying results. First-line therapy with corticosteroids at dosages ranging from 2 to 30 mg/kg/day resulted in improved hematological parameters in 10% to 30% of subjects within days of starting therapy without affecting tumor size.[4] IFN alone or in combination with steroids resulted in resolution of coagulopathy and tumor regression in approximately 40% of subjects.[4] However, the significant risk of irreversible neurotoxicity (spastic diplegia) in young infants treated with IFN has tempered its use.[24] VCR is emerging as a safe and effective treatment for KMP. In one series all 15 subjects treated with VCR as frontline therapy, either alone or in combination with other agents, experienced improved coagulation and hematologic parameters. 13 of these patients showed significant reductions in tumor size in response to VCR therapy.[25]

Despite cure of KMP, most patients remain with a large residual tumor after medical or surgical therapies.[13] These quiescent tumors can progress, often resulting in pain, functional impairment, and in rare instances, a late relapse of KMP.[13,26] Significant late effects in this population highlight the need for long-term follow-up and a better understanding of the unique biology of KHE to facilitate the development of new (targeted) therapies resulting in more complete resolution of the underlying malignancy.

SUMMARY

KMP is a rare condition with potentially fatal complications. It is associated with the vascular tumors KHE and TA and occurs most commonly in young infants. Treatment of KMP and the underlying malignancy requires a multidisciplinary team that can provide coordinated care over many years. Improvement in outcome will only be achieved through consensus on treatment guidelines and an improved understanding of the unique biology of this rare entity.

REFERENCES

1. Kasabach HH, Merritt KK. Capillary hemangioma with extensive purpura. Am J Dis Child 1940;59:1063–79.
2. Hall GW. Kasabach-Merritt syndrome: pathogenesis and management. Br J Haematol 2001;112(4):851–62.
3. Lyons LL, North PE, Mac-Moune Lai F, et al. Kaposiform hemangioendothelioma: a study of 33 cases emphasizing its pathologic, immunophenotypic, and biologic uniqueness from juvenile Hemangioma. Am J Surg Pathol 2004;28(5):559–68.
4. Sarkar M, Mulliken JB, Kozakewich HP, et al. Thrombocytopenic coagulopathy (Kasabach-Merritt phenomenon) is associated with Kaposiform hemangioendothelioma and not with common infantile hemangioma. Plast Reconstr Surg 1997;100(6):1377–86.
5. Enjolras O, Wassaf M, Mazoyer E, et al. Infants with Kasabach-Merritt syndrome do not have "true" hemangiomas. J Pediatr 1997;130(4):631–40.

6. Alvarez-Mendoza A, Lourdes TS, Ridaura-Sanz C, et al. Histopathology of vascular lesions found in Kasabach-Merritt syndrome: review based on 13 cases. Pediatr Dev Pathol 2000;3(6):556–60.
7. Shim WK. Hemangiomas of infancy complicated by thrombocytopenia. Am J Surg 1968;116(6):896–906.
8. Ryan C, Price V, John P, et al. Kasabach-Merritt phenomenon: a single centre experience. Eur J Haematol 2010;84(2):97–104.
9. Esterly N. Kasabach-Merritt syndrome in infants. J Am Acad Dermatol 1983;8(4):504–13.
10. Maceyko R, Camisa C. Kasabach-Merritt syndrome. Pediatr Dermatol 1991;8(2):133–6.
11. Zukerberg LR, Nickoloff BJ, Weiss SW. Kaposiform hemangioendothelioma of infancy and childhood. An aggressive neoplasm associated with Kasabach-Merritt syndrome and lymphangiomatosis. Am J Surg Pathol 1993;17(4):321–8.
12. Rodriquez V, Lee A, Witman PM, et al. Kasabach-Merritt phenomenon: case series and retrospective review of the mayo clinic experience. J Pediatr Hematol Oncol 2009;31(7):522–6.
13. Enjolras O, Mulliken B, Wassef M, et al. Residual lesions after Kasabach-Merritt phenomenon in 41 patients. J Am Acad Dermatol 2000;42(2):225–35.
14. Verheul HM, Panigrahy D, Flynn E, et al. Treatment of the Kasabach-Merritt syndrome with pegylated recombinant human megakaryocyte growth and development factor in mice: elevated platelet counts, prolonged survival, and tumor growth inhibition. Pediatr Res 1999;46(5):562–5.
15. Phillips WG, Marsden JR. Kasabach-Merritt syndrome exacerbated by platelet transfusion. J R Soc Med 1993;86:231–2.
16. Pampin C, Devillers A, Treguier C, et al. Intratumoral consumption of indium-111-labeled platelets in a child with splenic hemangioma and thrombocytopenia. J Pediatr Hematol Oncol 2000;22(3):256–8.
17. Seon KS, Jin CS, Gun YN, et al. Kasabach-Merritt syndrome: identification of platelet trapping in a tufted angioma by immunohistochemistry technique using monoclonal antibody to CD61. Pediatr Dermatol 1999;16(5):392–4.
18. Ortel T, Onorato J, Bedrosian C, et al. Antifibrinolytic therapy in the management of the kasabach merritt syndrome. Am J Hematol 1988;29(1):44–8.
19. Larsen E, Zinkham H, Eggleston C, et al. Kasabach-Merritt syndrome: therapeutic considerations. Pediatrics 1987;79:971–80.
20. Beaubien E, Ball N, Storwick G. Kaposiform hemangioendothelioma: a locally aggressive vascular tumor. J Am Acad Dermatol 1998;38(5):799–802.
21. Perez Payarols J, Pardo Masferrer J, Gomez Bellvert C. Treatment of life-threatening infantile hemangiomas with vincristine. N Engl J Med 1995;333:69–70.
22. Hu B, Lachman R, Phillips J, et al. Kasabach-Merritt syndrome-associated kaposiform hemangioendothelioma successfully treated with cyclophosphamide, vincristine, and actinomycin. D J Pediatr Hematol Oncol 1998;20(6):567–9.
23. Vin-Christian K, McCalmont T, Frieden I. Kaposiform Hemangioendothelioma: an aggressive, locally invasive vascular tumor that can mimic hemangioma of infancy. Arch Dematol 1997;133(12):1573–8.
24. Barlow C, Priebe C. Mulliken, Spastic diplegia as a complication of interferon Alfa-2a treatment of hemangiomas of infancy. J Pediatr 1998;133(3):527–30.
25. Haisley-Royster C, Enjolras O, Frieden I. Kasabach-Merritt phenomenon: a retrospective study of treatment with vincristine. J Pediatr Hematol Oncol 2002;24(6):459–62.
26. Ohtsuka T, Saegusa M, Yamakage S. Angioblastoma (Nakagawa) with hyperhidrosis, and relapse after a 10-year interval. Br J Dermatol 2000;143(1):223–4.

Vascular Malformations

Jennifer T. Huang, MD[a,b], Marilyn G. Liang, MD[a,b],*

KEYWORDS

- Vascular malformation • Capillary malformation
- Venous malformation • Lymphatic malformation
- Arteriovenous malformation • Glomuvenous malformations

Cutaneous vascular malformations are uncommon birthmarks that represent errors in vascular development and occur in approximately 0.3% to 0.5% of the population.[1] These lesions are much less common than infantile hemangiomas but are frequently confused with them. It is essential to properly diagnose these lesions because of their differences in morbidity, prognosis, and treatment.

CLASSIFICATION OF VASCULAR LESIONS

The classification of vascular anomalies has been hampered by the use of inaccurate terminology. Early classifications published by Virchow[2] characterized vascular lesions according to the vessel's pathologic appearance, dividing them into angiomas and lymphangiomas. The biologic behavior and natural history of the vascular lesions were not considered when classifying them. Thus, there was a tendency to identify any type of vascular anomaly as a hemangioma.

Mulliken and Glowacki[3] made great strides in clarifying this confusion when they published their landmark classification of vascular birthmarks in 1982, which grouped them into 2 major categories: hemangiomas and malformations. This classification has served as the foundation for the proper identification, investigation, and management of vascular birthmarks. Mulliken's biologic classification was modified slightly in 1996 to reflect new knowledge and the importance of other distinct types of vascular tumors, including the tumors that can cause Kasabach-Merritt phenomenon and others. The newer classification divided vascular birthmarks into *vascular tumors* and *vascular malformations*.[4] This classification of vascular anomalies has been widely

a Department of Dermatology, Harvard Medical School, c/o Massachusetts General Hospital, 55 Fruit Street, Bartlett 616, Boston, MA 02114, USA
b Dermatology Program, Children's Hospital Boston, 300 Longwood Avenue, Boston, MA 02115, USA
* Corresponding author. Dermatology Program, Children's Hospital Boston, 300 Longwood Avenue, Boston, MA 02115.

Pediatr Clin N Am 57 (2010) 1091–1110
doi:10.1016/j.pcl.2010.08.003
0031-3955/10/$ – see front matter © 2010 Elsevier Inc. All rights reserved.

adopted by clinicians and is the accepted classification of the International Society for the Study of Vascular Anomalies(ISSVA) (**Table 1**).

Although there are several types of vascular tumors, hemangiomas represent the overwhelming number of vascular tumors encountered by pediatricians. Hemangiomas are differentiated from vascular malformations by their clinical appearance, histopathologic features, and biologic behavior. Pediatricians should be most knowledgeable about differentiating hemangiomas from vascular malformations based on their clinical presentation. Hemangiomas are found to be more common in girls , whereas vascular malformations have an equal sex distribution. The natural course of hemangiomas involves rapid proliferation for the first several months of life with subsequent spontaneous regression, often leaving fibrofatty deposition, overlying anetoderma, and telangiectasias. Vascular malformations are often recognized at birth and grow proportionately with the child, with many becoming more prominent at puberty. In challenging cases, histopathologic evaluation, including immunohistochemical markers as well as radiologic studies, can further help to distinguish these two types of vascular anomalies (**Table 2**).[5–8] Despite these differences, the use of confusing nomenclature persists in the literature.

Vascular malformations can be further subdivided into groups based on vessel type and flow characteristics. Capillary, venous, and lymphatic malformations (LM) are slow-flow lesions, and arteriovenous malformations (AVM) and fistulae are fast-flow lesions. Combined lesions may also occur (see **Table 1**). Each type of vascular malformation is discussed in this article.

CAPILLARY MALFORMATIONS

Capillary malformations (CM), including fading capillary stains and port-wine stains, are among the most common vascular malformations affecting the skin (**Fig. 1**). True CM (the non-fading type) occur in approximately 3 of 1000 infants, are present

Table 1 Vascular anomalies' ISSVA/Mulliken classification 1996	
Vascular Tumors	**Vascular Malformations**
Infantile hemangioma	Simple
Congenital hemangioma (RICH, NICH)	Slow-flow
Pyogenic granuloma	Capillary (C) malformation
Tufted angioma	Lymphatic (L) malformation
Kaposiform hemangioendothelioma	Venous (V) malformation
Hemangiopericytoma	Glomuvenous malformation
	Fast-flow
	Arterial (A) malformation
	Combined
	Slow-flow
	LVM
	CLVM
	CVM
	Fast-flow
	AVM
	CM-AVM
	AVF

Abbreviations: AV, arteriovenous; F, fistula; M, malformation; NICH, non-involuting congenital hemangioma; RICH, rapidly involuting congenital hemangioma.

Table 2
Differentiating hemangiomas from vascular malformations

Characteristic	Infantile Hemangioma	Vascular Malformation
Age of Occurrence and Course	Infancy and childhood	Persistent if untreated
Sex Prevalence (Girl/Boy)	3–9:1	1:1
Natural History	Rapid growth followed by spontaneous regression	Proportional growth
Treatment	Spontaneous involution, pharmacologic treatment, surgery, lasers	Lasers, sclerotherapy, surgery

at birth, and are equally common in the male and female sex. They usually arise sporadically; however, familial cases in association with AVM have been described.[9]

Clinical Characteristics

A CM is usually noted at birth but may initially be misdiagnosed as a bruise or erythema from birth trauma. In young infants, CM may be pale pink macules and patches. They may present in small focal areas or involve an entire limb or portion of the face. Single or multiple lesions may occur. CM may arise on any surface of the skin but are frequently present on the head and neck area. When they are located on the head, they may extend to the lips, gingiva, or oral mucosa. Parents may note that the CM is somewhat darker in the immediate newborn period and lightens slightly in the first few weeks of life. This might be secondary to the higher hemoglobin concentration present in the immediate newborn period.[10]

The natural history of CM vary according to their anatomic location. The terms salmon patch, angel's kiss, stork bite, nevus simplex, and vascular stain are used to describe a subset of CM that are very common and located on the central face or nape of the neck. They are sometimes termed fading capillary stains rather than true CM, because these lesions typically lighten significantly or disappear early in life.[1] Some, often those located on the nape of the neck, persist into adulthood without significant darkening. Commonly used terms, such as angel's kiss, help to convey the benign nature of these common birthmarks to parents. Sometimes, it may prove difficult to differentiate a fading capillary stain located on the eyelid from true CM, infantile

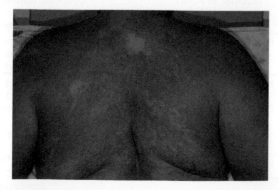

Fig. 1. Large CM.

Table 3
Vascular malformations and their associated syndromes

Vascular Malformation	Syndromes/Inheritance/Genes	Comments
CM	Sturge-Weber Inheritance/gene unidentified	CM in V1>V2 distribution Ipsilateral leptomeningeal angiomatosis Presents with seizures Ipsilateral glaucoma
	Phakomatosis pigmentovascularis Inheritance/gene unidentified	CM Epidermal nevus Dermal melanocytosis Nevus anemicus and/or nevus spilus
	Beckwith Wiedemann Inheritance unidentified Mutations in KIP2, H19, LIT1 OMIM#130650	Facial CM of midforehead, glabella, or upper eyelids Omphalocele Macrosomia Macroglossia
	Macrocephaly-CM Inheritance/gene unidentified	CM of central face Reticulated CM on trunk/extremities Macrocephaly Facial or limb asymmetry Somatic overgrowth
	Proteus Inheritance/gene unidentified OMIM#176920	Occasional CM Progressive overgrowth Epidermal nevus Cerebriform connective tissue nevus, often on soles
VM	Blue rubber bleb nevus Inheritance/gene unidentified	Cutaneous and gastrointestinal VM Risk of gastrointestinal hemorrhage
	Multiple cutaneous and mucosal VM Autosomal dominant Activating mutation in TIE2 OMIM#600195	Cutaneous and mucosal VM May have visceral VM
	GVMs Autosomal dominant Mutation in glomulin OMIM#138000	Multiple GVM No systemic involvement or associated findings reported
	Maffucci Inheritance unidentified Mutation in PTHR1 OMIM#166000	VM more common on hands and feet Dyschondroplasia Enchondromas Risk of chondrosarcoma
LM	Gorham Inheritance/gene unidentified	Most likely cutaneous LM Diffuse progressive osteolysis resulting in pathologic fractures
CLVM	Klippel-Trenaunay Inheritance/gene unidentified CLOVE Inheritance/gene unidentified	CLVM involving extremity (leg most common) Hyperplasia of soft tissue and bone Truncal CLVM Congenital lipomas Scoliosis Enlarged bony structures without progressive overgrowth

(continued on next page)

Table 3 (continued)		
Vascular Malformation	**Syndromes/Inheritance/Genes**	**Comments**
AVM	Parkes-Weber	AVM of extremity
	Inheritance unidentified	Hyperplasia of soft tissue and
	Mutation in RASA1	bone
	OMIM#608355	
	CM-AVM	Multiple cutaneous CM
	Autosomal dominant	Cutaneous, subcutaneous,
	Mutation in RASA1	intraosseous, and/or cerebral
	OMIM#608354	AVM
	Hereditary hemorrhagic	AVM of lungs, liver,
	telangiectasia	gastrointestinal tract, and/or
	Autosomal dominant	brain
	Multiple mutations including:	Mucocutaneous telangiectasias
	Type 1: endoglin	Presents commonly with epistaxis
	OMIM#187300	Risk of visceral hemorrhage
	Type 2: ALK1	
	OMIM#600376	
	Coexisting juvenile	
	polyposis:	
	SMAD4	
	OMIM#175050	
	Bannayan-Riley-Ruvalcaba	AVM or AVF
	Inheritance unidentified	Macrocephaly
	Mutation in PTEN	Lipomas
	OMIM#153480	Genital lentigines
	Cobb	Association of CM with underlying
	Inheritance/gene unidentified	spinal AVM

Abbreviations: AVF, arteriovenous fistula; CLOVE, congenital lipomatous overgrowth, vascular malformations, and epidermal nevi; CLVM, capillary-lymphatic-venous malformation; GVM, glomuvenous malformation; OMIM, online Mendelian inheritance in man; VM, venous malformation.

hemangioma precursors, or minimally proliferative infantile hemangiomas; so, reassessment within the first few months of life may be required.

In contrast to these benign fading stains, as the patient matures, true facial CM may become darker, more violaceous, and thicker and develop blebs. These lesions are also known as port-wine stains and may also be associated with underlying soft-tissue hypertrophy.

Associated Findings and Syndromes

CM of the skin may occur in association with other congenital malformations, including underlying vascular anomalies or other structural abnormalities of ectodermal origin, such as bony or soft-tissue hyperplasia or atrophy, or neurologic defects. In particular, limb CM may be associated with congenital hypertrophy of underlying bone and soft tissue.

Some of these associated anomalies occur with more frequency and have been assigned various eponyms (**Table 3**). The most common of these is Sturge-Weber syndrome, a neuroectodermal syndrome characterized by a CM in the V1 (and sometimes V2) distribution of the trigeminal nerve, ipsilateral leptomeningeal angiomatosis, and glaucoma (**Fig. 2**). Seizures are the most common neurologic feature, often present within the first year of life, and they may be difficult to control.

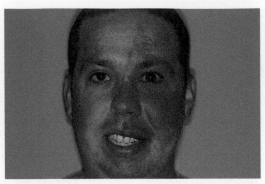

Fig. 2. CM status post pulsed dye laser treatment in Sturge-Weber syndrome. (with permission from the patient.)

Macrocephaly-CM syndrome is characterized by CM on the central face and macrocephaly, which can be progressive. Reticulated CM may also be located on the trunk or extremities. Often, these patients also have structural brain abnormalities. Other minor features include developmental delay, limb abnormalities, and joint or skin laxity.[11] Proteus syndrome is a rare overgrowth syndrome that is characterized by progressive overgrowth (typically of a limb), epidermal nevi, and connective tissue nevi. CM are reported in some patients.[12]

A less well-recognized anomaly associated with CM is underlying spinal dysraphism, which may occur in the lumbar region, and in the neck area when the CM is associated with an underlying mass or pit.[13,14] A retrospective review has suggested that the combination of two or more midline cutaneous lesions is highly suggestive of occult spinal dysraphism in children. However, this study did not include other types of birthmarks.[15] The significance of these CM as a marker of spinal dysraphism when they occur in isolation is unclear and controversial, and specific evidence-based guidelines regarding screening spinal evaluations with magnetic resonance imaging (MRI) or ultrasonography do not exist.

CM may also be associated with other vascular malformations. The development of blebs and hyperkeratotic areas within CM on the extremities is virtually always seen in association with a lymphatic and/or venous malformation (VM). As mentioned previously, familial cases of CM in association with cutaneous, subcutaneous, and/or cerebral AVM, so-called CM-AVM, have been reported. Finally, CM overlying the spinal cord may be a cutaneous sign of an underlying spinal AVM and has been called Cobb syndrome. CM-AVM and Cobb syndrome are discussed in more detail in the AVM section of this article.

Diagnosis and Management

CM are diagnosed based on their appearance and behavior. Cutaneous erythema overlying a deeper AVM or a minimally proliferative infantile hemangioma may mimic a CM. For suspected cases, Doppler ultrasound evaluation is helpful but not always diagnostic in differentiating an arteriovenous fistula or shunt from a CM.[8]

Once the diagnosis of CM is established, the patient should be evaluated for the presence of underlying vascular malformations and associated congenital anomalies. Multiple different subspecialists can care for CM and other vascular malformations. Referral to a vascular anomalies center, where multidisciplinary care is provided, is advised for further evaluation and treatment of CM.

The flashlamp-pumped pulsed dye laser (PDL) is the treatment of choice for CM. The most commonly used lasers use a wavelength that selectively targets oxyhemo-globin (577, 585, 595 nm) resulting in intravascular coagulation, as well as pulse durations that limit destruction and heat dissipation to the CM vasculature without causing damage to the surrounding structures in the epidermis or dermis. The current generation of PDLs uses epidermal cooling devices that minimize damage to the surrounding structures and lessens discomfort associated with treatment. Response to treatment is variable, with some investigators reporting good response in as many as 80% of treated subjects.[16] Parents should be counseled that complete disappearance of the lesion is unlikely; however, cosmetically acceptable results occur in most patients after multiple treatments.[17,18] Some patients who have initially undergone successful lightening using the traditional PDL may show re-darkening of their lesions several years after successful therapy.[19] Although other laser types and light sources, such as the alexandrite, neodymium-doped yttrium-aluminium-garnet (Nd:YAG), and intense pulsed light, and photodynamic therapy have been used, the efficacy and associated risks are still uncertain.[20] Thus, PDL remains the standard of care for laser treatment of CM.

Laser treatment is often used in conjunction with local or general anesthesia. Younger patients may require general anesthesia to treat extensive CM.[21] Treatment during early childhood is desirable to minimize the psychosocial impact of a significant congenital malformation.[22,23] In some situations, smaller lesions on older children may be treated without anesthesia. Sessions are scheduled every 6 to 8 weeks over the course of several months to years, depending on the size and responsiveness of the lesion. CM located on the central face and limb are generally less responsive to laser therapy than those on other regions of the face, neck, and trunk.[24] There is no minimum age required. It has been suggested that younger patients may respond better, with more significant lightening, than older patients. This observation remains controversial, because some authors found no evidence that treatment of CM with PDL in early childhood is more effective than treatment later in the first decade of life.[25–27]

VM

VM are slow-flow vascular malformations that are typically noted at birth (**Fig. 3**). They are slowly expanding vascular birthmarks composed of anomalous dilated venous channels. Mucocutaneous VM are uncommon, but when present, they may have

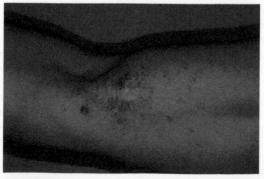

Fig. 3. VM on the arm post-biopsy.

significant consequences. These lesions usually arise sporadically, but familial VM can occur and are inherited in an autosomal dominant manner.

VM have previously been called venous angioma, cavernous angioma, cavernous hemangioma, and phlebangioma in the medical literature. The term cavernous hemangioma is particularly confusing and should be avoided, because it often leads to the mislabeling of lesions as infantile hemangioma. Glomuvenous malformations (GVM), a distinct subtype of VM, are also discussed later.

Clinical Characteristics

VM are usually noted at birth but, in some cases, may not become evident until the child matures. They typically become more prominent over time; parents and patients often report the most dramatic changes within the first decades of life with fewer changes during adulthood. VM present as soft blue masses that may be easily compressed with gentle pressure. They become more prominent with activity or if the affected area is held in a dependent position. They are usually blue to purple, and they do not demonstrate any increase in warmth or thrill to palpation. If these finding are present, a mixed AVM should be suspected.

VM may arise on the skin or the mucosal surfaces. They may be small focal lesions or larger and cover a significant portion of the head and neck or extremity. Cervicofacial VM are worrisome, because they may extend into deeper structures, which may be difficult to appreciate on initial examination without radiologic studies. Large facial VM may lead to deformation of the underlying or adjacent structures, such as the tongue, teeth, and bones. Orofacial VM may cause bleeding, airway obstruction, and speech and dental abnormalities.

VM located on the arms and legs may also be localized or diffuse. Extensive limb VM occurring without an overlying CM may be confused with Klippel-Trenaunay syndrome. VM on the limbs may cause functional difficulties by involving the skeletal muscle and joint spaces. When they are located in the deeper subcutaneous tissues, they may go unnoticed until the patient develops pain or swelling, sometimes following trauma later in life.[28]

VM, particularly when located on the limbs, are commonly associated with episodes of pain that are usually an indication of larger lesions and/or muscle involvement. Other complications of VM include phlebolith formation and localized intravascular coagulopathy (LIC).[29] LIC has previously been mistaken for the thrombocytopenic coagulopathy associated with vascular tumors (Kasabach-Merritt phenomenon) but is a distinct entity.[30] VM-associated LIC causes pain and may result in severe bleeding if it is not recognized before surgical procedures. The hallmark of this coagulopathy is an elevated D-dimer level and variable fibrinogen level. This finding is so common that some authors have suggested that it may be used to help differentiate VM from other types of vascular malformations, such as a GVM and LM, which do not show elevated D-dimer levels. The management of LIC in the setting of VM remains somewhat controversial, with some groups advocating anticoagulation with low–molecular-weight heparin and others with low-dose aspirin depending on the severity of the findings.[31–34]

GVM, previously known as glomangioma, is a type of VM that is distinct from typical VM. Lesions arise in infancy or later in life and have a variable clinical presentation. They may present as small blue papules or as larger pebbly plaques covering a larger area of the skin surface (the latter known as congenital plaque-type GVM). They are typically more firm and less compressible than typical VM. Patients may report pain with prolonged compression. Histologic examination, when performed, demonstrates anomalous venous channels lined by cuboidal glomus cells. GVM are often familial and are inherited in an autosomal dominant manner. However, the presentation within affected families may be variable, with some children demonstrating the extensive congenital plaque-type GVM and other affected family members showing trivial involvement of the skin surface.[35] GVM are more frequently confined to the skin and subcutaneous tissues compared with typical VM and are not associated with LIC. Isolated lesions are most commonly present on the upper extremities, particularly the nail beds (glomus tumors). Multiple lesions are more suggestive of an inherited form of GVM. A family history and examination of other family members can be very helpful in supporting the diagnosis of GVM.[36,37]

Associated Findings and Syndromes

Most cases of VM are sporadic without associated findings. However, there are 2 rare syndromes with clinical features that include VM: blue rubber bleb nevus syndrome (Bean syndrome) and Maffucci syndrome. Blue rubber bleb nevus syndrome is characterized by the presence of cutaneous and gastrointestinal VM; these patients are at risk of severe gastrointestinal bleeding. The VM of blue rubber bleb nevus syndrome typically become more apparent with maturity. There have also been familial cases of cutaneous and mucosal VM reported. Genetic analysis of these families has mapped an activating mutation in the gene that encodes for the kinase domain of the endothelial cell receptor TIE2.[38,39] Although the first cases did not report gastrointestinal involvement, subsequent families with this mutation have had VM of the gastrointestinal tract.[40] Sporadic cases of VM have also been linked to a somatic mutation in TIE2, providing some insight into the pathogenesis of VM and, perhaps, future therapeutic strategies.[41] Maffucci syndrome is a rare disorder characterized by the combination of dyschondroplasia resulting in enchondromas and VM most commonly on the distal extremities.

Multiple GVM are often inherited in an autosomal dominant fashion and linked to a loss-of-function mutation in glomulin. GVM are typically confined to the skin and subcutaneous tissues. Systemic involvement or other associated findings are not reported.[42]

Diagnosis and Management

MRI is the most useful imaging modality to confirm the diagnosis of VM and to define the extent of involvement in the skin and subcutaneous tissues.[8,43] Doppler ultrasonography is also helpful to confirm that the lesion is not high-flow and to assess the patency of the deep venous system.

A multidisciplinary approach to therapy is important for the management of VM, and many medical centers now have multispecialty teams and clinics that work to coordinate the care of these often complex VM. In many cases, management is not curative. The management goals depend on the location of the VM and the extent of involvement in the skin. Some lesions are managed with supportive care without surgical intervention. It is recommended that a coagulation profile including D-dimers be obtained at the time of diagnosis, when patients complain of pain and before any form of active treatment is undertaken.[31] VM may be treated with Nd:YAG laser therapy, sclerotherapy, surgical excision, endovenous laser therapy, or combination therapy.[44–46] Small localized lesions may be managed with a single modality. Sclerotherapy and Nd:YAG laser therapy are often used on mucosal lesions. Laser therapy with the Nd:YAG may be helpful in areas in which there are concerns about the possibility of superficial scarring following sclerotherapy.[45] The traditional PDL that is used for the treatment of CM is ineffective for the treatment of VM. In larger lesions, surgical excision alone may be difficult because of the size and location of the lesions and the risk of bleeding. Recurrences are reported following these treatment modalities. A combination of sclerotherapy, surgical excision, and laser treatment may be necessary in large cervicofacial lesions.[47] Ultrasound-guided endovenous laser therapy, typically used for treatment of varicose veins, has been explored recently, with success.[48,49]

Treatment of trunk and limb VM is difficult and patients are usually managed conservatively. As discussed previously, patients with larger lesions have a high incidence of chronic LIC.[28,30,31] Patients with extensive limb lesions should be instructed from childhood in the proper use of compression garments; however, compliance may be a challenge. Compression garments help to decrease the discomfort associated with the lesion, protect the overlying skin, limit swelling, and improve LIC. Active intervention with a surgical modality (laser therapy, sclerotherapy, or excisional surgery) may be considered in small and/or shallow lesions. Surgical excision may also be used to debulk very large VM.

It is now recognized that GVM respond differently to treatment than typical VM. Sclerotherapy may be less effective and patients may report increased discomfort with the use of compression garments.[36,50] Surgical excision or laser therapy may be considered for isolated lesions.

LM

LM are developmental anomalies of the lymphatic system that manifest as diffuse abnormalities in lymphatic drainage/flow or anomalous collections of lymphatic vessels. Interpretation of the literature on this topic has been challenging, because of the use of many different terms to describe various different lymphatic anomalies.[51–55]

LM follow different patterns and may be classified as primary or secondary and localized or diffuse (**Table 4**). The term lymphedema is used to describe a diffuse lymphatic anomaly, often of the limbs. Acquired (also called secondary) lymphedema is caused by disruption of the normal lymphatic drainage, which may be caused by trauma, infection, or scarring. Primary lymphedema occurs less frequently, may be seen in the pediatric population (**Fig. 4**), and can be an isolated anomaly in association with other disorders (eg, Noonan and Turner syndromes). Primary lymphedema, which is not associated with these well-characterized genetic syndromes, is traditionally classified

Table 4	
Classification of lymphatic malformations	
Diffuse (Lymphedema)	**Localized**
Primary	Macrocystic
Congenital familial (Nonne-Milroy disease)	Microcystic
Lymphedema praecox (Meige disease)	
Lymphedema tarda	
Associated syndromes	
Lymphedema distichiasis	
Turner syndrome	
Noonan syndrome	
Acquired	
Infections	
Surgery	
Radiotherapy	

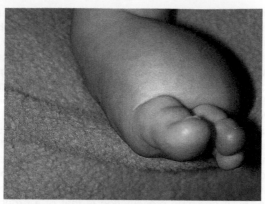

Fig. 4. Primary lymphedema.

into groups based on the age at onset: hereditary lymphedema type I (primary congenital lymphedema, Nonne-Milroy disease), hereditary lymphedema type II (lymphedema praecox, late-onset hereditary lymphedema, or Meige disease), and a later-onset form, lymphedema tarda.[55] Milroy disease is inherited in an autosomal dominant manner and is caused by mutations in the FMS-like tyrosine kinase-4 gene (FLT4) that encodes for the vascular endothelial growth factor receptor 3.[56] This disorder presents at birth with lymphedema of the lower extremities. Lymphedema praecox is a more common form of lymphedema, which typically presents during adolescence with lymphedema of one or both legs.

Lower-extremity lymphedema may also be seen in association with a double row of eyelashes, which is called lymphedema-distichiasis syndrome. This rare disorder is inherited in an autosomal dominant pattern and is associated with mutations in FOXC2.[57] The lymphedema associated with Turner syndrome and Noonan syndrome is believed to be caused by hypoplasia of the normal lymphatic system.[58–62]

Localized LM present during infancy or become apparent during childhood. These LM are often called lymphangiomas and are classified as macrocystic or microcystic lesions. LM arise as isolated lesions or in combination with other vascular malformations. Macrocystic LM of the head and neck are also called cystic hygromas. Lymphangioma circumscriptum is an older term used to describe microcystic LM with a superficial component. LM may be both microcystic and macrocystic, but it is useful to characterize these lesions because the size of the cysts may affect treatment and prognosis.

Clinical Characteristics

Most LM present at birth, with the remainder becoming evident within the first few years of life.[63] Several studies show no sex predilection , whereas others report a higher incidence in the male sex.[64–67]

Most macrocystic LM are present at birth and may be diagnosed on prenatal ultrasonography. They are often located on the neck and upper truncal area. In some patients, they present as isolated ill-defined subcutaneous masses that expand over time as the anomalous lymphatic channels become dilated. They may remain asymptomatic or cause localized pain. Large macrocystic LM located on the neck may be noted before birth and, in some cases, interfere with delivery.[68] Other complications include airway obstruction, feeding and speech difficulties, and recurrent infections within the LM.[69,70] Head and neck LM (macrocystic or combined micro/ macrocystic lesions) may also be associated with bony hypertrophy that may arise during early childhood. Progressive distortion of the mandible may occur in children with LM involving the tongue, oral cavity, and neck and lead to significant disfigurement.[70] Orbital LM, which may be mistaken for infantile hemangioma, can cause swelling, pain, proptosis, and visual compromise.[69] LM may also arise within the abdomen and lead to pain and distension and, in rare cases, symptoms of small bowel obstruction from volvulus.[70,71]

Microcystic LM are present at birth but may not become evident until later in childhood. Parents often note an area of swelling within the skin, with slight discoloration of the skin surface that may develop acutely. The seemingly sudden appearance of an LM is often secondary to infection or bleeding caused by trauma to the LM.[72] Microcystic LM may arise anywhere on the body but are often found on the proximal extremities and trunk (**Fig. 5**). A common presentation is that of a group of brown-to-tan papules, which may be mistaken for warts, overlying a localized or larger area of the skin. The papules may become hemorrhagic or crusted or develop black dots within them.[73] These superficial lesions usually represent the tip of the iceberg, giving the mistaken impression that they are well-circumscribed when, in reality, they are more diffusely distributed in the subcutaneous tissues. The most common symptom is recurrent oozing of clear fluid or blood. Secondary infection, skin erosions, and bleeding are frequently reported complications of microcystic LM. Squamous cell carcinoma has also been reported to arise within a long-standing microcystic LM.[74]

Associated Findings and Syndromes

LM may present in association with CM. Some authors suggest that angiokeratomas are examples of combined CM and LM.[1] Lymphatic anomalies are also a component of complex combined vascular malformations and may be seen in some patients with Klippel-Trenaunay syndrome (**Fig. 6**).

Diagnosis and Management

LM is usually suspected based on history and clinical features. However, imaging studies, including ultrasonography and MRI, confirm the diagnosis and delineate the extent of involvement within the subcutaneous tissues. As noted earlier, macrocystic LM (cystic hygroma) may be detected on prenatal ultrasonography and may be associated with polyhydramnios.[75–77]

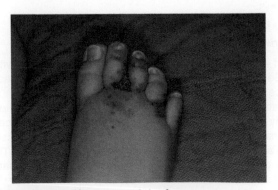

Fig. 5. Microcystic lymphatic malformation of the foot.

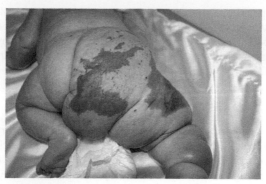

Fig. 6. Klippel-Trenaunay syndrome on the leg.

Management of LM needs to be individualized. Important factors to be considered when planning management include the size and location of the lesion, whether the lesion is microcystic or macrocystic, and whether it is associated with other anomalies. A multidisciplinary approach is needed, because a combination of therapies may be required. It is important to advise parents that complete removal of some types of LM is not possible. Bacterial superinfection is a common and important complication of LM and should be managed promptly. Guidance should be provided to parents regarding signs of infection, and they should be instructed to seek treatment promptly at the first signs of redness, sudden enlargement of the lesion, tenderness, or fever. Suspected secondary infection within an LM should be treated with systemic antibiotics that cover typical skin pathogens. Intravenous administration of antibiotics might be required; therefore, children with suspected minor infections who are initially placed on oral antibiotics should be monitored closely to make sure that they are improving with therapy.

Percutaneous sclerotherapy and excisional surgery may be used to manage LM. Various different sclerosing agents have been used to treat LM and may be more effective and easier to perform in patients with macrocystic rather than microcystic LM.[78] Surgical excision is pursued in some patients with localized circumscribed lesions. For larger lesions, complete excision may not be possible, and/or multiple procedures may be required. Postsurgical complications include wound infections, damage to surrounding structures, such as the facial nerve, and recurrence of the LM. Even lesions that appear to be completely excised at the time of surgery may show recurrences with rates as high as 27%. Partial excisions are associated with much higher recurrence rates; therefore, parents should be advised carefully before making a decision regarding this modality.[68,69,79] Nd:YAG laser and CO_2 lasers have been reported for the treatment of LM; however, as with other surgical modalities, recurrences are also common after treatment.[80,81]

CAPILLARY-LYMPHATIC-VENOUS MALFORMATIONS

Although most vascular malformations can be defined by the vessel type primarily involved, some are composed of a complex combination of multiple vessel types. These malformations are termed capillary-lymphatic-venous malformations (CLVM). CLVM may occur in isolation or as part of a syndrome. Klippel-Trenaunay syndrome is characterized by the triad of a CLVM of an extremity, venous varicosities, and hyperplasia of soft tissue and bone. In addition to orthopedic difficulties due to limb overgrowth, these patients are at risk of thrombophlebitis and coagulopathy. Congenital lipomatous overgrowth, vascular malformations, epidermal nevi (CLOVE) is a recently described syndrome characterized most commonly by truncal CLVM, congenital lipomas, scoliosis, and enlarged bony structures without progressive overgrowth.[82]

AVMS

AVMs are rare fast-flow vascular lesions composed of anomalous arterial and venous vessels connected directly to each other without an intervening capillary bed (**Fig. 7**). They are among the most challenging vascular lesions to diagnose in early childhood and often are not recognized as AVM until they become more fully developed with maturity.

Clinical Characteristics

AVM occur in the male and female sex with equal frequency. Approximately half are visible in the neonatal period, and others become apparent during childhood. These lesions are often mistaken for other types of vascular birthmarks, particularly CM. Periodic reassessment during childhood often provides clues (increased warmth to palpation, increasing prominence of vessels).

The Schobinger staging system has been used to describe 4 stages through which an AVM may progress.[83,84] Stage I AVM are pink patches or macules that often mimic a subtle CM. The presence of increased warmth or thrill to palpation suggests a high-flow component, which may be detected on Doppler ultrasonography. Stage I AVM are asymptomatic and often remain so until adolescence. Some AVM remain in this stage throughout a patient's lifetime. During stage II, the AVM become more prominent as the vessels within them become more dilated.[85] There is increased warmth to palpation and a thrill may be noted. Additional changes include prominent draining veins, and, in some cases, the skin may thicken and become more purple. In adults, the changes may mimic Kaposi sarcoma.[86-89] Progression from stage I to stage II is often noted at the time of puberty, following trauma or partial treatment of the AVM.[84] Stage III is characterized by destruction of deeper tissues, including bone, as well as pain and hemorrhage. Stage IV is characterized by cardiac compromise from increased blood flow.

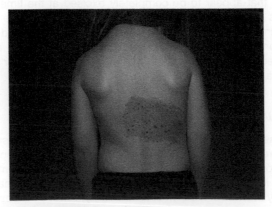

Fig. 7. AVM with multiple pyogenic granulomas.

Associated Findings and Syndromes

Familial cases of CM in association with AVM, known as CM-AVM, have been described and linked to an inactivating mutation in RASA1.[9,90] CM-AVM is inherited in an autosomal dominant fashion. These patients have multiple cutaneous CM as well as cutaneous, subcutaneous, intramuscular, intraosseous, and/or cerebral AVM.

Parkes Weber syndrome is characterized by the presence of an AVM on an extremity (which may mimic a CM), often with concomitant soft-tissue and bony hypertrophy. This syndrome was thought to be sporadic and nonhereditary until recently, when several cases were identified to also have a genetic mutation in RASA1.[91]

Another syndrome associated with AVM is hereditary hemorrhagic telangiectasia (HHT), also called Osler-Weber-Rendu syndrome. HHT is an autosomal dominant vascular disorder characterized by mucocutaneous telangiectasias, bleeding diathesis, and visceral AVM. AVM can occur in the lungs, liver, gastrointestinal tract, and central nervous system, may result in massive visceral hemorrhage, and are significantly responsible for the morbidity and mortality related to this disease.[92] Some cases of HHT are associated with juvenile polyposis.[93]

Cobb syndrome, also called cutaneomeningospinal angiomatosis, consists of the association of a CM on the midline of the back with an intraspinal AVM. The cutaneous lesion is located along the midline of the back, with the corresponding intraspinal AVM within a segment or two of the involved dermatome.[92] Although rare, recognizing this association is essential for diagnosis and prompt treatment of a potentially debilitating spinal cord lesion.

Diagnosis and Management

AVM are diagnosed by clinical findings and radiologic features. The diagnosis may be delayed for years if the lesion remains quiescent. Doppler ultrasonography and MR techniques are often used to support the diagnosis in suspected cases of AVM.[8] The differential diagnosis of AVM includes other vascular malformations, vascular neoplasms, and in rare cases, other neoplasms. Pain, increased warmth, and bleeding episodes provide clues to the diagnosis but are not specific to AVM. The presence of a bruit on auscultation or with bedside Doppler ultrasonography supports the diagnosis of AVM. Once the diagnosis is established, it is important to obtain a careful family history for vascular birthmarks and, when possible, examine other affected family members, because it has become recognized that there is great phenotypic variability within families with CM-AVM syndrome. The management of AVM is challenging, and complete eradication of the lesion may not be possible. A multidisciplinary approach with physicians who have experience with AVM management is essential, because partial treatment, such as partial surgical excision or embolization, may result in a recurrence that is more problematic than the initial lesion. Quiescent stage I AVM that are not impairing an important function or causing disfigurement are often managed conservatively with close monitoring. Significant pain, bleeding, or ulceration and enlargement of the malformation are often indications for treatment. The timing of intervention is controversial and lesion-dependent. Some reports suggest that treatment of stage I lesions has a higher success rate than of later-stage AVM.[84] When treatment is indicated, a multidisciplinary approach, including preoperative embolization and complete surgical resection, is often necessary for the management of AVM.

SUMMARY

Vascular malformations are rare but important skin disorders of which pediatricians should be aware. It is essential to distinguish these lesions from the more common infantile hemangioma. Although fading capillary stains may be managed by pediatricians with parental education and reassurance, the diagnosis and management of most other vascular malformations require assistance from subspecialists and, optimally, in a multidisciplinary setting, such as a vascular anomaly center. Therefore, this article strives to provide the pediatrician with an armamentarium of vocabulary regarding vascular malformations, to better communicate with their patients and medical colleagues when discussing the clinical characteristics, diagnostic criteria, and treatment options of these lesions.

REFERENCES

1. Boon LM, Vikkula M. Vascular malformations. In: Wolff K, Goldsmith LA, Katz SI, et al, editors. Fitzpatrick's dermatology in general medicine. New York: McGraw Hill; 2008. p. 1651–66.
2. Virchow R, editor. Die krankhaften Geschwülste. Berlin: A. Hirschwald; 1863. p. 456–61.
3. Mulliken JB, Glowacki J. Hemangiomas and vascular malformations in infants and children: a classification based on endothelial characteristics. Plast Reconstr Surg 1982;69(3):412–20.
4. Enjolras O, Mulliken JB. Vascular tumors and vascular malformations (new issues). Adv Dermatol 1997;13:375–423.
5. Takahashi K, Mulliken JB, Kozakewich HP, et al. Cellular markers that distinguish the phases of hemangioma during infancy and childhood. J Clin Invest 1993; 93(6):2357–64.
6. North PE, Waner M, Mizeracki A, et al. A unique microvascular phenotype shared by juvenile hemangiomas and human placenta. Arch Dermatol 2001;137(5): 559–70.
7. Burrows PE, Mulliken JB, Fellows KE, et al. Childhood hemangiomas and vascular malformations: angiographic differentiation. Am J Roentgenol 1983; 141(3):483–8.
8. Dubois J, Garel L. Imaging and therapeutic approach of hemangiomas and vascular malformations in the pediatric age group. Pediatr Radiol 1999;29(12): 879–93.
9. Eerola I, Boon LM, Mulliken JB, et al. Capillary malformation-arteriovenous malformation, a new clinical and genetic disorder caused by RASA1 mutations. Am J Hum Genet 2003;73(6):1240–9.
10. Cordoro KM, Speetzen LS, Koerper MA, et al. Physiologic changes in vascular birthmarks during early infancy: mechanisms and clinical implications. J Am Acad Dermatol 2009;60(4):669–75.
11. Wright DR, Frieden IJ, Orlow SJ, et al. The misnomer "macrocephaly-cutis marmorata telangiectactica congenital syndrome": report of 12 new cases and support for revising the name to macrocephaly-capillary malformations. Arch Dermatol 2009;145(3):287–93.
12. Biesecker L. The challenges of Proteus syndrome: diagnosis and management. Eur J Hum Genet 2006;14(11):1151–7.
13. Davis DA, Cohen PR, George RE. Cutaneous stigmata of occult spinal dysraphism. J Am Acad Dermatol 1994;31(5 Pt 2):892–6.
14. Enjolras O, Boukobza M, Jdid R. Cervical occult spinal dysraphism: MRI findings and the value of a vascular birthmark. Pediatr Dermatol 1995;12(3):256–9.
15. Guggisberg D, Hadj-Rabia S, Vinet C, et al. Skin markers of occult spinal dysraphism in children: a review of 54 cases. Arch Dermatol 2004;140(9):1109–15.

16. Reyes BA, Geronemus R. Treatment of port-wine stains during childhood with the flashlamp-pumped pulsed dye laser. J Am Acad Dermatol 1990;23(6 Pt 1): 1142–8.
17. Garden JM, Polla LL, Tan OT. The treatment of port-wine stains by the pulsed dye laser. Analysis of pulse duration and long term therapy. Arch Dermatol 1988; 124(6):889–96.
18. Goldman MP, Fitzpatrick RE, Ruiz-Esparza J. Treatment of port-wine stains (capillary malformation) with the flashlamp-pulsed dye laser. J Pediatr 1993;122(1): 71–7.
19. Orten SS, Waner M, Flock S, et al. Port-wine stains. An assessment of 5 years of treatment. Arch Otolaryngol Head Neck Surg 1996;122(11):1174–9.
20. McGill DJ, MacLaren W, Mackay IR. A direct comparison of pulsed dye, alexandrite, KTP, and Nd-YAG lasers and IPL in patients with previously treated capillary malformations. Lasers Surg Med 2008;40(6):390–8.
21. Grevelink JM, White VR, Bonoan R, et al. Pulsed laser treatment in children and the use of general anesthesia. J Am Acad Dermatol 1997;37(1):75–81.
22. Lanigan SW, Cotterill JA. Psychological disabilities amongst patients with port-wine stains. Br J Dermatol 1989;121(2):209–15.
23. Malm M, Carlberg M. Port-wine stain- a surgical and psychological problem. Ann Plast Surg 1988;20(6):512–6.
24. Renfro L, Geronemus RG. Anatomical differences of port-wine stains in response to treatment with the pulsed dye laser. Arch Dermatol 1993;129(2):182–8.
25. Ashinoff R, Geronemus RG. Flashlamp-pumped pulsed dye laser for port-wine stains in infancy: earlier versus later treatment. J Am Acad Dermatol 1991; 24(3):467–72.
26. Van der Horst CM, Koster PH, deBorgie CA, et al. Effect of the timing of treatment of port-wine stains with the flash-lamp-pumped pulsed-dye laser. N Engl J Med 1998;338(15):1028–33.
27. Ackermann G, Hartmann M, Scherer K, et al. Correlations between light penetration into skin and the therapeutic outcome following laser therapy of port-wine stains. Lasers Med Sci 2002;17(2):70–8.
28. Enjolras O, Ciabrini D, Mazoyer E, et al. Extensive pure venous malformations in the upper or lower limb: a review of 27 cases. J Am Acad Dermatol 1997;36(2 Pt 1): 219–25.
29. Enjolras O, Mulliken JB. The current management of vascular birthmarks. Pediatr Dermatol 1993;10(4):311–33.
30. Mazoyer E, Enjolras O, Laurian C, et al. Coagulation abnormalities associated with extensive venous malformations of the limbs: differentiation from Kasabach-Merritt syndrome. Clin Lab Haematol 2002;24(4):243–51.
31. Mazoyer E, Enjolras O, Bisdorff A, et al. Coagulation disorders in patients with venous malformation of the limbs and trunk: a case series of 118 patients. Arch Dermatol 2008;144(7):861–7.
32. Dompmartin A, Acher A, Thibon P, et al. Association of localized intravascular coagulopathy with venous malformations. Arch Dermatol 2008;144(7): 873–7.
33. Dompmartin A, Ballieux F, Thibon P, et al. Elevated D-dimer level in the differential diagnosis of venous malformations. Arch Dermatol 2009;145(11):1239–44.
34. Maguiness S, Koerper M, Frieden I. Relevance of D-dimer testing in patients with venous malformations. Arch Dermatol 2009;145(11):1321–4.
35. Mallory SB, Enjolras O, Boon LM, et al. Congenital plaque-type glomuvenous malformations presenting in childhood. Arch Dermatol 2006;142(7):892–6.

36. Boon LM, Mulliken JB, Enjolras O, et al. Glomuvenous malformation (glomangioma) and venous malformation: distinct clinicopathologic and genetic entities. Arch Dermatol 2004;140(8):971–6.
37. Brouillard P, Ghassibé M, Penington A, et al. Four common glomulin mutations cause two thirds of glomuvenous malformations ("familial glomangiomas"): evidence for a founder effect. J Med Genet 2005;42(2):e13.
38. Vikkula M, Boon LM, Carraway KL, et al. Vascular dysmorphogenesis caused by an activating mutation in the receptor tyrosine kinase TIE2. Cell 1996;87(7): 1181–90.
39. Calvert JT, Riney TJ, Kontos CD, et al. Allelic and locus heterogeneity in inherited venous malformations. Hum Mol Genet 1999;8(7):1279–89.
40. Gallione CJ, Pasyk KA, Boon LM, et al. A gene for familial venous malformations maps to chromosome 9p in a second large kindred. J Med Genet 1995;32(3):197–9.
41. Limaye N, Wouters V, Uebelhoer M, et al. Somatic mutations in angiopoietin receptor gene TEK cause solitary and multiple sporadic venous malformations. Nat Genet 2009;41(1):118–24.
42. Brouillard P, Boon LM, Mulliken JB, et al. Mutations in a novel factor, glomulin, are responsible for glomuvenous malformations ('glomangiomas'). Am J Hum Genet 2002;70(4):866–74.
43. Rak KM, Yakes WF, Ray RL, et al. MR imaging of symptomatic peripheral vascular malformations. AJR Am J Roentgenol 1992;159(1):107–12.
44. Dubois JM, Sebag GH, DeProst G, et al. Soft-tissue venous malformations in children: percutaneous sclerotherapy with Ethibloc. Radiology 1991;180(1):195–8.
45. Scherer K, Waner M. Nd:YAG lasers (1,064 nm) in the treatment of venous malformations of the face and neck: challenges and benefits. Lasers Med Sci 2007;22(2):119–26.
46. Garzon MC, Huang JT, Enjolras O, et al. Vascular malformations: Part I. J Am Acad Dermatol 2007;56(3):353–70.
47. Glade RS, Richter GT, James CA, et al. Diagnosis and management of pediatric cervicofacial venous malformations: retrospective review from a vascular anomalies center. Laryngoscope 2010;120(2):229–35.
48. Sidhu MK, Perkins JA, Shaw DWW, et al. Ultrasound-guided endovenous diode laser treatment of congenital venous malformations: preliminary experience. J Vasc Interv Radiol 2005;16(6):879–84.
49. Berber O, Holt P, Hinchliffe R, et al. Endovenous therapy for the treatment of congenital venous maformations. Ann Vasc Surg 2010;24(3):415.e13–7.
50. Mounayer C, Wassef M, Enjolras O, et al. Facial "glomangiomas": large facial venous malformations with glomus cells. J Am Acad Dermatol 2001;45(2):239–45.
51. Kinmonth JB, editor. The lymphatics. London: Arnold; 1982. p. 116–27.
52. Hilliard RI, McKendry JB, Phillips MJ. Congenital abnormalities of the lymphatic system: a new clinical classification. Pediatrics 1990;86(6):988–94.
53. Bruna J, Miller AJ, Beninson J. A universally applicable clinical classification of lymphedema. Angiology 1999;50(3):189–92.
54. Williams HB. Vascular neoplasms. Clin Plast Surg 1980;7(3):397–411.
55. Witte MH, Witte CL. Lymphangiogenesis and lymphologic syndromes. Lymphology 1986;19(1):21–8.
56. Evans AL, Bell R, Brice G, et al. Identification of eight novel VEGFR-3 mutations in families with primary lymphoedema. J Med Genet 2003;40(9):697–703.
57. Fang J, Dagenais SL, Erickson RP, et al. Mutations in FOXC2 (MFH-1), a forkhead family transcription factor, are responsible for the hereditary lymphedema-distichiasis syndrome. Am J Hum Genet 2000;67(6):1382–8.

58. Lowenstein EJ, Kim KH, Glick SA. Turner's syndrome in dermatology. J Am Acad Dermatol 2004;50(5):767–76.
59. Vittay P, Bosze P, Gaal M, et al. Lymph vessel defects in patients with ovarian dysgenesis. Clin Genet 1980;18(5):387–91.
60. Hall JG, Gilchrist DM. Turner syndrome and its variants. Pediatr Clin North Am 1990;37(6):1421–40.
61. Katz VL, Kort B, Watson WJ. Progression of nonimmune hydrops in a fetus with Noonan syndrome. Am J Perinatol 1993;10(6):417–8.
62. Witt DR, Hoyme HE, Zonana J, et al. Lymphedema in Noonan syndrome: clues to pathogenesis and prenatal diagnosis and review of the literature. Am J Med Genet 1987;27(4):841–56.
63. Redondo P. [Classification of vascular anomalies (tumours and malformations). Clinical characteristics and natural history]. An Sist Sanit Navar 2004;27(Suppl 1): 9–25 [in Spanish].
64. Ninh TN, Ninh TX. Cystic hygroma in children: a report of 126 cases. J Pediatr Surg 1974;9(2):191–5.
65. Saijo M, Munro IR, Mancer K. Lymphangioma. A long-term follow-up study. Plast Reconstr Surg 1975;56(6):642–51.
66. Brock ME, Smith RJ, Parey SE, et al. Lymphangioma. An otolaryngologic perspective. Int J Pediatr Otorhinolaryngol 1987;14(2–3):133–40.
67. Hancock BJ, St-Vil D, Luks FI, et al. Complications of lymphangiomas in children. J Pediatr Surg 1992;27(2):220–40 [discussion: 224–6].
68. Padwa BL, Hayward PG, Ferraro NF, et al. Cervicofacial lymphatic malformation: clinical course, surgical intervention, and pathogenesis of skeletal hypertrophy. Plast Reconstr Surg 1995;95(6):951–60.
69. Greene AK, Burrows PE, Smith L, et al. Periorbital lymphatic malformation: clinical course and management in 42 patients. Plast Reconstr Surg 2005;115(1):22–30.
70. Lin JI, Fisher J, Caty MG. Newborn intraabdominal cystic lymphatic malformations. Semin Pediatr Surg 2000;9(3):141–5.
71. Traubici J, Daneman A, Wales P, et al. Mesenteric lymphatic malformation associated with small-bowel volvulus - two cases and a review of the literature. Pediatr Radiol 2002;32(5):362–5.
72. Peachey RD, Lim CC, Whimster IW. Lymphangioma of skin. A review of 65 cases. Br J Dermatol 1970;83(5):519–27.
73. Darmstadt GL. Perianal lymphangioma circumscriptum mistaken for genital warts. Pediatrics 1996;98(3 Pt 1):461–3.
74. Wilson GR, Cox NH, McLean NR, et al. Squamous cell carcinoma arising within congenital lymphangioma circumscriptum. Br J Dermatol 1993;129(3):337–9.
75. Chervenak FA, Isaacson G, Blakemore KJ, et al. Fetal cystic hygroma. Cause and natural history. N Engl J Med 1983;309(14):822–5.
76. McAlvany JP, Jorizzo JL, Zanolli D, et al. Magnetic resonance imaging in the evaluation of lymphangioma circumscriptum. Arch Dermatol 1993;129(2): 194–7.
77. Davies D, Rogers M, Lam A, et al. Localized microcystic lymphatic malformations—ultrasound diagnosis. Pediatr Dermatol 1999;16(6):423–9.
78. Shiels WE, Kang DR, Murakami JW, et al. Percutaneous treatment of lymphatic malformations. Otolaryngol Head Neck Surg 2009;141(2):219–24.
79. Fageeh N, Manoukian J, Tewfik T, et al. Management of head and neck lymphatic malformations in children. J Otolaryngol 1997;26(4):253–8.
80. Tasar F, Tumer C, Sener BC, et al. Lymphangioma treatment with Nd-YAG laser. Turk J Pediatr 1995;37(3):253–6.

81. Haas AF, Narurkar VA. Recalcitrant breast lymphangioma circumscriptum treated by UltraPulse carbon dioxide laser. Dermatol Surg 1998;24(8):893–5.
82. Sapp JC, Turner JT, van de Kamp JM, et al. Newly delineated syndrome of congenital lipomatous overgrowth, vascular malformations, and epidermal nevi (CLOVE syndrome) in seven patients. Am J Med Genet A 2007;143(24):2944–58.
83. Enjolras O, Logeart I, Gelbert F, et al. [Malformations artérioveineuses: étude de 200 cas]. Ann Dermatol Venereol 1999;127(1):17–22 [in French].
84. Kohout MP, Hansen M, Pribaz JJ, et al. Arteriovenous malformations of the head and neck: natural history and management. Plast Reconstr Surg 1998;102(3):643–54.
85. Young AE. Arteriovenous malformations. In: Mulliken JB, Young AE, editors. Vascular birthmarks: hemangiomas and malformations. Philadelphia: WB Saunders; 1988. p. 228–45.
86. Earhart RN, Aeling JA, Nuss DD, et al. Pseudo-Kaposi sarcoma. A patient with arteriovenous malformation and skin lesions simulating Kaposi sarcoma. Arch Dermatol 1974;110(6):907–10.
87. Amon RB. Letter: arteriovenous malformation resembling Kaposi sarcoma. Arch Dermatol 1975;111(12):1656–7.
88. Brenner S, Ophir J, Krakowski A, et al. Kaposi-like arteriovenous malformation and angiodermatitis (pseudo-Kaposi). Cutis 1982;30(2):240–2, 247, 255–6.
89. Larralde M, Gonzalez V, Marietti R, et al. Pseudo-Kaposi sarcoma with arteriovenous malformation. Pediatr Dermatol 2001;18(4):325–7.
90. Boon LM, Mulliken JB, Vikkula M. RASA1: variable phenotype with capillary and arteriovenous malformations. Curr Opin Genet Dev 2005;15(3):265–9.
91. Revencu N, Boon LM, Mulliken JB, et al. Parkes Weber syndrome, vein of Galen aneurysmal malformation, and other fast-flow vascular anomalies are caused by RASA1 mutations. Hum Mutat 2008;29(7):959–65.
92. Paller AS, Mancini AJ. Vascular disorders of infancy and childhood. In: Paller AS, Mancini AJ, editors. Hurwitz clinical pediatric dermatology. Philadelphia: Elsevier; 2006. p. 322–31.
93. Gallione CJ, Repetto GM, Legius E, et al. A combined syndrome of juvenile polyposis and hereditary haemorrhagic telangiectasia associated with mutations in MADH4(SMAD4). Lancet 2004;363(9412):852–9.

Genetics and Syndromes Associated with Vascular Malformations

Kelly Duffy, PhD

KEYWORDS

- Vascular malformation • Genetic syndromes
- Genetic testing • Vascular anomaly • Overgrowth

Historically, vascular malformations were not thought to be the result of genetic abnormalities because most of those presenting clinically are sporadic. However, research in this field has expanded over the last decade, leading to the identification of genetic defects responsible for several inherited forms of vascular malformations and associated syndromes, which has shed light on the pathogenesis of sporadic lesions. This advancement in the field has not only enhanced diagnostic capabilities but has also improved our understanding of the potential role of complex genetic mechanisms in vascular malformation development.

It is important for pediatricians to recognize genetically determined vascular malformations and their associated syndromes because there are several disease-specific risks, including various forms of cancer, coagulopathies, pulmonary embolism, and cardiac overload. Genetic testing may be extremely useful for clinical management, screening, and treatment decision making but should be performed only with proper education of the patients and their families. The clinical characteristics of vascular malformations are discussed in the article by Marilyn Liang elsewhere in this issue; this article focuses on genetic contributions to vascular malformations, vascular malformations in the context of syndromes, and the tests that are available.

CURRENT KNOWLEDGE

Vascular malformations are localized structural defects of the vasculature, named after the type of vessel affected.[1] Although some forms of vascular malformations are inherited, a majority occurs sporadically. It is postulated that vascular

Dermatology Department, Pediatric Dermatology, Medical College of Wisconsin, 8701 Watertown Plank Road, Milwaukee, WI 53226, USA
E-mail address: kduffy@mcw.edu

Pediatr Clin N Am 57 (2010) 1111–1120
doi:10.1016/j.pcl.2010.07.001
0031-3955/10/$ – see front matter © 2010 Elsevier Inc. All rights reserved.

pediatric.theclinics.com

Table 1
Mutations identified in vascular anomalies and associated syndromes

Malformation	Mode of Inheritance	Locus	Gene	Mutations	Pathways/Functions
Capillary malformation	Sporadic	—	—	—	—
Capillary malformation-arteriovenous malformation	Autosomal dominant	5q13-22	RASA1	Loss of function	Ras-MAPK pathways; cell growth, proliferation, motility, survival
Cerebral cavernous malformation	Sporadic	—	—	—	Adaptor proteins, integrin β1 pathway, cell adhesion, migration
	Autosomal dominant	7q11-22 7p13 3q26.1 3q26.3-27.2	KRIT1 Malcavernin PDCD10	Loss of function, somatic second hits	
Venous malformation	Sporadic	9p21	TIE2/TEK	Somatic, gain of function	Tyrosine kinase receptor, EC proliferation, migration, survival; smooth muscle cell recruitment; vascular sprouting and maturation
Glomuvenous malformation	Autosomal dominant	1p21-22	GLMN	Loss of function, somatic second hit	TGFβ, HGF pathways; protein synthesis; smooth muscle cell differentiation
Cutaneomucosal venous malformation	Autosomal dominant	9p21	TIE2/TEK	Gain of function	Tyrosine kinase receptor; smooth muscle cell recruitment, vascular sprouting, EC proliferation and migration
Lymphatic malformation	Sporadic	—	—	—	—
Primary lymphedema (Milroy disease)	Sporadic Autosomal dominant/recessive	5q35.3	VEGFR3/FLT4	De novo, loss of function Loss of function	Tyrosine kinase receptor; angiogenesis, lymphangiogenesis, EC proliferation, migration, survival

Syndrome	Inheritance	Locus	Gene	Mutation	Pathway/Function
Lymphedema distichiasis	Sporadic; Autosomal dominant	16q24.3	FOXC2	De novo, loss of function; Loss of function	VEGF, Notch, Insulin, TGFβ pathways; transcription factor, angiogenesis
Arteriovenous malformation	Sporadic	—	—	—	—
Hereditary hemorrhagic telangiectasia	Autosomal dominant	9q33-34	ENG	Loss of function	TGFβ, MAPK pathways; EC hypoxia survival, migration, proliferation; vascular organization
Multifocal lymphangio-endotheliomatosis with thrombocytopenia	Sporadic	—	—	—	—
Blue rubber bleb nevus syndrome	Sporadic	—	—	—	—
Maffucci syndrome	Sporadic	—	—	—	—
Klippel-Trénaunay syndrome	Sporadic	—	—	—	—
PTEN hamartoma tumor syndrome	Autosomal dominant	10q23	PTEN	Loss of function, loss of heterozygosity	PI3K/Akt pathway; cellular proliferation, migration, survival, angiogenesis
Congenital lipomatosis overgrowth, vascular malformation, epidermal nevus, scoliosis syndrome	Sporadic	—	—	—	—
Sturge-Weber syndrome	Sporadic	—	—	—	—
Parkes-Weber syndrome (solitary capillary malformation)	Sporadic	—	—	—	—
Parkes Weber syndrome (multifocal capillary malformation)	Sporadic; Inherited[a]	5q13-22	RASA1	De novo, loss of function; Loss of function	Ras-MAPK pathways; cell growth, proliferation, motility, survival
Proteus syndrome	Sporadic	—	—	—	—

Abbreviations: EC, endothelial cell; HGF, hepatocyte growth factor; MAPK, mitogen-activated protein kinase; PI3K, phosphoinositide-3 kinase; PTEN, phosphatase and tensin homologue on chromosome 10; TGF, transforming growth factor; VEGF, vascular endothelial growth factor.

[a] Mode of inheritance could not be determined from reporting study.[7]

malformations and some associated syndromes are the result of a somatic mutation creating a mosaic clinical phenotype, in which 2 genetically distinct populations of cells exist within the same individual.[2] These malformations are present at birth, tend to grow proportionately with the child, and do not regress spontaneously. The malformations vary greatly in number, size, and location, and can also occur in the context of syndromes.[3] **Table 1** summarizes current knowledge regarding genetic contributions to vascular malformations and syndromes with a significant vascular malformation component.

Capillary Malformations

Capillary malformations typically occur as sporadic, solitary, cutaneous lesions with unknown cause. Some capillary malformations are also associated with arteriovenous malformations (CM-AVMs), characterized by small, multifocal, capillary malformations surrounded by a pale halo (**Fig. 1**).[4,5] CM-AVM is associated with loss-of-function mutations in the RASA1 gene inherited in an autosomal dominant manner.[6] Approximately 30% of affected individuals have deeper, fast-flow lesions such as arteriovenous malformations (AVMs) or arteriovenous fistulas (AVFs) in addition to the capillary malformations.[7] It is noteworthy that more than 80% of these fast-flow lesions are located in the head and neck regions either intra- or extracranially.[7] Of

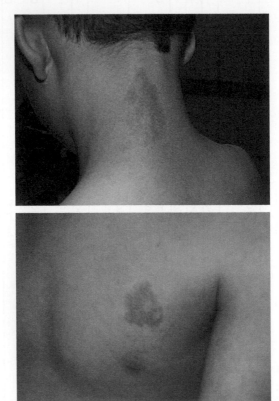

Fig. 1. Child with multifocal capillary malformations (*top*) and AVM, associated with mutation of the RASA1 gene. Note the pale halo on the skin surrounding the capillary malformations.

the 30% of individuals with AVM or AVF, about one-third have Parkes-Weber syndrome, characterized by underlying tissue overgrowth of the affected limb.[7] The phenotypic variability and the fact that not all individuals with RASA1 mutations have associated fast-flow lesions and overgrowth suggest that additional mutational events are required for CM-AVM and Parkes-Weber syndrome.

Cerebral Cavernous Malformations

Cerebral cavernous malformations often occur in the brain, retina, and spinal cord, but are sometimes accompanied by hyperkarotic cutaneous lesions.[8,9] It has been reported that 4 genetic loci are inherited in an autosomal dominant manner in cerebral cavernous malformations, of which 3 have genes carrying loss-of-function mutations (see **Table 1**), and the fourth locus was suggested by linkage to a region of 3q.[10–14] Hundreds of mutations have been identified in these loci, most resulting in loss of function; double hits have also been reported in some cases[15,16] suggesting paradominance as a potential inheritance model.

Venous Malformations

About 95% of venous malformations are solitary lesions of variable size that occur sporadically in nature.[17] Small, multifocal, venous malformations that are found on the skin and mucosa may sometimes follow an autosomal dominant pattern of inheritance. These lesions are called cutaneomucosal venous malformations, and are caused by mutations in the TEK gene that encodes the tyrosine kinase receptor TIE2.[17–20] Approximately 50% of sporadic venous malformations were found to contain somatic mutations in TIE2,[18] suggesting that inherited forms may also require a somatic alteration of the second allele to develop the vascular lesions. Proper diagnosis of these lesions is important because they are often associated with coagulopathies, and individuals can experience pain resulting from the presence of phleboliths within the abnormal vessels. Another type of venous malformation is the glomuvenous malformation, which is characterized by multifocal nodular lesions and the presence of glomus cells around the distended vascular channels. Glomuvenous malformations are caused by loss-of-function mutations in the glomulin gene that are inherited in an autosomal dominant manner,[5] although the identification of double-hit mutations may indicate the possibility of paradominant inheritance.[5]

Lymphatic Malformations

Lymphatic malformations can be localized or diffuse; they are thought to be the result of developmental defects during embryonic lymphangiogenesis,[21] and are only known to occur sporadically. Although the etiology of lymphatic malformations is unknown, genetic studies on lymphedema have identified crucial factors involved in lymphatic development that can serve as candidates for future study (see **Table 1**).

Combined Malformations

AVMs are high-flow, sporadic lesions that can be localized or diffuse. AVMs can occur in association with other vascular phenotypes such as CM-AVM and Parkes-Weber syndrome, discussed earlier, among others. Hereditary hemorrhagic telangiectasia is an autosomal dominant disorder characterized by cutaneomucosal telangiectasias, epistaxis, and often AVMs. At least 4 loci have been associated with hereditary hemorrhagic telangiectasia, with mutations in 2 genes, endoglin and activin receptor-like kinase.[22–25] Other combined malformations include capillary-venous, lymphatic-venous, and capillary-lymphatic-venous lesions, though their causes are unknown.

Table 2
Syndromes with a predominant vascular malformation component

Syndrome	Associated Phenotype	Vascular Component
Sturge-Weber syndrome	Facial capillary malformation and vascular malformation of eye (typically glaucoma) and/or brain	Capillary malformation of face; conjunctiva, episclera, retina, and/or choroids; vascular malformation of the brain consists of hypoplastic cortical vessels associated with enlarged and tortuous leptomeningeal vessels and often dilated deep venous vessels
Klippel-Trénaunay syndrome	Superficial vascular stain of the skin in association with soft tissue and bony hypertrophy of the affected limb and varicose veins with or without deep venous anomalies	Capillary, lymphatic, venous, or combined slow-flow malformations
Proteus syndrome	Soft tissue and bony hypertrophy of the hands and feet, hemihypertrophy, exostosis, cranial hyperostosis, visceral hamartomas including lipomas, vascular anomalies, and epidermal nevi	Capillary, lymphatic, venous, or combined slow-flow malformations
Parkes Weber syndrome	Overgrowth of an extremity linked to the presence of an AVM with multiple arteriovenous fistulas along the affected extremity addition to a cutaneous red stain	Capillary malformation and AVM or fistula
PTEN hamartoma tumor syndrome	Macrocephaly, macrosomia at birth, lipomas, hamartomatous intestinal polyposis, variable degrees of developmental delay, and pigmented macules on the glans penis, mucocutaneous lesions, such as facial trichilemmomas, cobblestone-like papules on the oral mucosa, acral keratosis, and various papillomatous lesions	Capillary malformations, sometimes multifocal AVMs
CLOVES syndrome	Congenital lipomatous overgrowth, vascular malformations, epidermal nevi, and scoliosis	Capillary, lymphatic, venous, or combined slow-flow malformations
Maffucci syndrome	Enchondromas and vascular anomalies	Venous malformations within bone and on hands is common

Syndromes

Although many syndromes have a known genetic basis, such as Parkes-Weber syndrome with multifocal capillary malformations and those that make up the phosphatase and tensin homologue (PTEN) hamartoma tumor syndrome, the genetic contributions to most syndromes associated with vascular malformations are not fully understood. Such syndromes include Sturge-Weber, Klippel-Trénaunay, Maffucci, blue rubber bleb nevus, CLOVES (congenital lipomatosis overgrowth, vascular malformation, epidermal nevus, and scoliosis) syndrome, and proteus (**Table 2**). The PTEN hamartoma tumor syndrome is a constellation of hamartomatous syndromes that are phenotypically variable but have germline mutations in the PTEN tumor suppressor gene.

WHEN TO CONSIDER GENETIC TESTING

As a pediatrician, it is important to consider atypical genetic mechanisms (**Box 1**) in the scope of vascular malformations and associated syndromes. Because most vascular malformations are visible on the skin, the pediatrician can use that accessibility to gather important diagnostic clues that may indicate the presence of other malformations. Identification of a lesion or syndrome that suggests a genetic cause can lead to a more accurate diagnosis and improved disease management and treatment. Patients who should be considered for genetic testing include, but are not limited to, those with multifocal vascular lesions, those with a family history of birthmarks, and those with vascular stains and any associated over- or undergrowth (**Box 2**).

GENETIC TESTS AVAILABLE

Over the past few years there has been a significant increase in the number and scope of genetic tests used to confirm a vascular malformation or related syndrome

---

Box 1
Definitions

Somatic mutation

   An acquired postzygotic mutation; not heritable

Germline mutation

   A mutation in a germ cell that is inherited

Mosaicism

   The presence of 2 genetically distinct cell populations in the same individual

Sporadic

   Spontaneously occurring, not inherited

Double hit/Second hit

   An inherited mutation of one gene allele with subsequent somatic mutation of the second allele

Paradominance

   A theory of inheritance in which individuals heterozygous for a mutation are phenotypically normal, but those who acquire a somatic second hit manifest the disease

---

Box 2
Questions to consider if vascular malformation or associated syndrome is suspected

Question	Potential Implication
Is the lesion solitary or multifocal?	Multifocal lesions tend to occur in the heritable forms of vascular malformations/syndromes for which genetic testing may be available to assist in accurate diagnosis; multifocal lesions also suggest there may be visceral lesions
What color is the lesion and does the color ever change?	Color can assist in the clinical assessment of the type of vessel involvement in the lesion; abnormalities of different vessel types can lead to distinct risk factors
Is it painful? If so, is it localized pain? Is it constant pain or does it only occur under certain circumstances (during activity, only in morning, and so forth)	Pain can indicate many things depending on the type of malformation. The associated venous malformations and syndromes are at an increased risk of developing blood clots, which can cause significant pain in the lesion and present risk for clot to travel elsewhere in the body. This complication can happen any time; however, it is most commonly experienced in the morning. Patients with Klippel-Trénaunay and CLOVES syndromes are at a higher risk for developing pulmonary embolisms. Lymphatic malformations are often painful because of lymphedema and pressure on the surrounding tissue and infection
Does the lesion ever swell? Does swelling only occur under certain circumstances?	Lymphatic malformations often result in lymphedema, which can lead to pain and infection and often occurs in the lower extremities after long periods of standing, and in the head and neck region
Is there a family history of lesions or birthmarks?	Family history indicates inheritance, and genetic testing may assist in accurate diagnosis
Has the lesion been there since birth?	Vascular malformations are congenital and most are visible at or shortly after birth
Has the lesion grown over time or stayed about the same size?	Growing lesions can lead to further complications and may require more aggressive treatment
Is there a history of glaucoma, headaches, or seizures?	Glaucoma, headaches, and/or seizures in the context of a facial capillary malformation (port-wine stain) suggest the presence of Sturge-Weber syndrome
Are there are any major or minor growth abnormalities associated with the lesion?	Numerous growth abnormalities are associated with vascular malformations, from slight discrepancies to severe and distorting asymmetric overgrowth

---

diagnosis. **Table 3** describes genetic tests available at present. Not all genetic tests are commercially available for clinical use; some are only available for research purposes. Proper education of patients and their families by the physician and a genetic counselor prior to genetic testing, and proper interpretation of results is essential for appropriate decision making. As intense research efforts continue to result in the development of new diagnostic genetic tests, it is imperative that

Table 3
Genetic tests currently available

Gene Test	Test Availability	Methods
RASA1	Clinical and research	Analysis of entire coding region; sequence analysis
KRIT1	Clinical	Analysis of entire coding region; sequence analysis; targeted mutation analysis; linkage analysis
Tie2/TEK	Research	Mutation screening
GLMN	Research	Mutation screening
VEGFR3/FLT4	Clinical and research	Analysis of entire coding region; sequence analysis
FOXC2	Clinical and research	Analysis of entire coding region; sequence analysis
ENG	Clinical and research	Analysis of entire coding region; sequence analysis; deletion/duplication analysis
PTEN	Clinical and research	Bidirectional sequence analysis of coding exons, splice sites, and core promoter region; duplication/deletion analysis

Data from http://www.ncbi.nlm.nih.gov/sites/GeneTests.

physicians continually update their knowledge on what is available in an effort to provide the most options for their patients.

REFERENCES

1. Brouillard P, Vikkula M. Vascular malformations: localized defects in vascular morphogenesis. Clin Genet 2003;63(5):340–51.
2. Happle R. Lethal genes surviving by mosaicism: a possible explanation for sporadic birth defects involving the skin. J Am Acad Dermatol 1987;16(4): 899–906.
3. Mulliken JB, Young AE. Vascular birthmarks: hemangiomas and malformations. Philadelphia: Saunders; 1998.
4. Boon LM, Mulliken JB, Vikkula M. RASA1: variable phenotype with capillary and arteriovenous malformations. Curr Opin Genet Dev 2005;15(3):265–9.
5. Brouillard P, Vikkula M. Genetic causes of vascular malformations. Hum Mol Genet 2007;16(Spec No. 2):R140–9.
6. Eerola I, Boon LM, Mulliken JB, et al. Capillary malformation-arteriovenous malformation, a new clinical and genetic disorder caused by RASA1 mutations. Am J Hum Genet 2003;73(6):1240–9.
7. Revencu N, Boon LM, Mulliken JB, et al. Parkes Weber syndrome, vein of Galen aneurysmal malformation, and other fast-flow vascular anomalies are caused by RASA1 mutations. Hum Mutat 2008;29(7):959–65.
8. Labauge P, Enjolras O, Bonerandi JJ, et al. An association between autosomal dominant cerebral cavernomas and a distinctive hyperkeratotic cutaneous vascular malformation in 4 families. Ann Neurol 1999;45(2):250–4.
9. Eerola I, Plate KH, Spiegel R, et al. KRIT1 is mutated in hyperkeratotic cutaneous capillary-venous malformation associated with cerebral capillary malformation. Hum Mol Genet 2000;9(9):1351–5.

10. Laberge-le Couteulx S, Jung HH, Labauge P, et al. Truncating mutations in CCM1, encoding KRIT1, cause hereditary cavernous angiomas. Nat Genet 1999;23(2):189–93.
11. Sahoo T, Johnson EW, Thomas JW, et al. Mutations in the gene encoding KRIT1, a Krev-1/rap1a binding protein, cause cerebral cavernous malformations (CCM1). Hum Mol Genet 1999;8(12):2325–33.
12. Liquori CL, Berg MJ, Siegel AM, et al. Mutations in a gene encoding a novel protein containing a phosphotyrosine-binding domain cause type 2 cerebral cavernous malformations. Am J Hum Genet 2003;73(6):1459–64.
13. Bergametti F, Denier C, Labauge P, et al. Mutations within the programmed cell death 10 gene cause cerebral cavernous malformations. Am J Hum Genet 2005;76(1):42–51.
14. Liquori CL, Berg MJ, Squitieri F, et al. Low frequency of PDCD10 mutations in a panel of CCM3 probands: potential for a fourth CCM locus. Hum Mutat 2006; 27(1):118.
15. Kehrer-Sawatzki H, Wilda M, Braun VM, et al. Mutation and expression analysis of the KRIT1 gene associated with cerebral cavernous malformations (CCM1). Acta Neuropathol 2002;104(3):231–40.
16. Gault J, Shenkar R, Recksiek P, et al. Biallelic somatic and germ line CCM1 truncating mutations in a cerebral cavernous malformation lesion. Stroke 2005;36(4): 872–4.
17. Vikkula M, Boon LM, Carraway KL 3rd, et al. Vascular dysmorphogenesis caused by an activating mutation in the receptor tyrosine kinase TIE2. Cell 1996;87(7): 1181–90.
18. Limaye N, Wouters V, Uebelhoer M, et al. Somatic mutations in angiopoietin receptor gene TEK cause solitary and multiple sporadic venous malformations. Nat Genet 2009;41(1):118–24.
19. Pagon RA, Bird TC, Dolan CR, et al, editors. GeneReviews [internet]. Seattle (WA): University of Washington; 1993–2008.
20. Calvert JT, Riney TJ, Kontos CD, et al. Allelic and locus heterogeneity in inherited venous malformations. Hum Mol Genet 1999;8(7):1279–89.
21. Blei F. Congenital lymphatic malformations. Ann N Y Acad Sci 2008;1131:185–94.
22. McAllister KA, Grogg KM, Johnson DW, et al. Endoglin, a TGF-beta binding protein of endothelial cells, is the gene for hereditary haemorrhagic telangiectasia type 1. Nat Genet 1994;8(4):345–51.
23. Johnson DW, Berg JN, Baldwin MA, et al. Mutations in the activin receptor-like kinase 1 gene in hereditary haemorrhagic telangiectasia type 2. Nat Genet 1996;13(2):189–95.
24. Cole SG, Begbie ME, Wallace GM, et al. A new locus for hereditary haemorrhagic telangiectasia (HHT3) maps to chromosome 5. J Med Genet 2005;42(7):577–82.
25. Bayrak-Toydemir P, McDonald J, Akarsu N, et al. A fourth locus for hereditary hemorrhagic telangiectasia maps to chromosome 7. Am J Med Genet A 2006; 140(20):2155–62.

Patterned Pigmentation in Children

James Treat, MD

KEYWORDS

- Patterned pigmentation • Segmental pigmentary disorder
- Pigmentary mosaicism • Hypermelanosis • Hypomelanosis
- Blaschkoid pigmentation • Segmental nevus depigmentosus
- Incontinentia pigmenti

Patterned pigmentation describes a phenotype in which the skin has lighter or darker shades in a particular pattern. The skin pigmentation can either be isolated or signal an underlying disorder with systemic manifestations. The most commonly recognized patterns of cutaneous pigmentation are those following lines of Blaschko (which can be thin or broad), checkerboard pattern, and phyloid or leaf pattern (**Fig. 1**).[1] Blaschko's lines mark the embryonic migration of ectodermal cells, with both melanocytes and keratinocytes arising from the ectoderm. Blaschko's lines are more wavy and whorled than the straight bands of dermatomes, which follow the distribution of cutaneous sensory nerves. Pigmentary demarcation lines can often be seen vertically oriented on the upper anterior arms and lower abdomen in dark-skinned patients, and are normal physiologic patterns that do not signify a disorder.

If a genetic error leads to a distinct set of cells that has a darker or lighter phenotype, Blaschko's lines become visible as a line of darker or lighter pigmentation along that cell and its progeny's migration path. The term pigmentary mosaicism is often used to describe these patterns. In some situations, the genetic error resulting in dyspigmentation may also result in abnormalities that are not isolated to the skin.[2] This term implies two separate cell lines in the same person. Whether mosaicism is the cause of the patterned pigmentation in all patients is unknown.[3] Pigmentary mosaicism may manifest as areas of hypopigmentation or hyperpigmentation in an individual; however, the areas that represent the "baseline" skin color may be difficult to distinguish from the areas of dyspigmentation in an individual with extensive pigment mosaicism (**Fig. 2**).

Hypomelanosis of Ito (HI) and linear and whorled nevoid hypermelanosis (LWNH) are syndromes that are classically described as being associated with pigmentary

Funding Support: None.
Department of Pediatrics, Section of Dermatology, University of Pennsylvania School of Medicine, Children's Hospital of Philadelphia, 3550 Market Street, 2nd Floor Dermatology, Philadelphia, PA 19104, USA
E-mail address: treat@email.chop.edu

Pediatr Clin N Am 57 (2010) 1121–1129
doi:10.1016/j.pcl.2010.07.007
0031-3955/10/$ – see front matter © 2010 Elsevier Inc. All rights reserved.

pediatric.theclinics.com

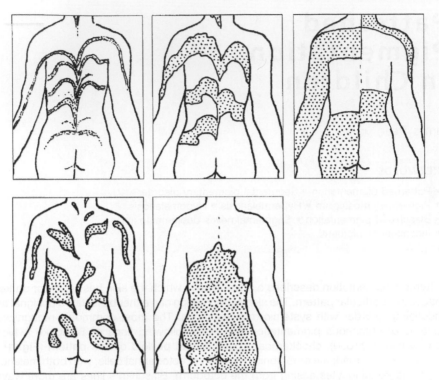

Fig. 1. Patterns of cutaneous mosaicism. (*From* Happle R. Mosaicism in human skin: understanding the patterns and mechanisms. Arch Dermatol 1993;129(11):1460–70; with permission.)

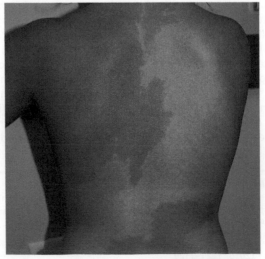

Fig. 2. Patterned pigmentation. The areas that represent the baseline pigmentation are difficult to determine in this patient.

mosaicism. Not all patients with patterned pigmentation have extensive involvement. Hogeling and Frieden[4] recently described a subset of patients with block-like and unilateral hypo- or hyperpigmentation (similar to the checkerboard or phyloid patterns described by Happle[1]) who rarely have associated anomalies, using the term *segmental pigmentary disorder* (SegPD) to describe the condition. This term was originally described by Metzker and colleagues.[5]

Paller[6] proposed that the earlier in development a genetic error occurs, the more tissues it is likely to affect. Therefore, the more widespread a pigmentary anomaly is, the more likely it is associated with underlying systemic abnormalities. Unfortunately, the terminology is confusing because the genotype–phenotype correlations and exact pathophysiology are still being investigated, but attempting to separate patients with very low risk for systemic anomalies (SegPD) will help avoid unnecessary workup.

MECHANISMS OF MOSAICISM

The most readily recognized pattern of mosaicism in humans is the programmed inactivation that occurs of one X chromosome in women with XX karyotype (lyonization).[7] This ability to inactivate aberrant or potentially dangerous genetic material on one X chromosome essentially allows women to pick the best genetic material. This selection confers protection from life-threatening genetic conditions carried on the X chromosome, which are often lethal in men who are forced to use their only copy of the X chromosome (eg, incontinentia pigmenti).

Happle[8] originally suggested that abnormalities within lines of Blaschko resulted from lyonization within these cells and their progeny as they migrated. Probably many different types of genetic aberrations can lead to pigmentary mosaicism. Some patients with patterned hyperpigmentation or hypopigmentation (LWNH) phenotype and HI phenotype) have been described with a balanced translocation of an autosomal chromosome to an X chromosome, and disruption of Xp11 was described in earlier case series of patients with HI.[9,10]

More recently Taibjee and colleagues[2] proposed that X;autosome translocations lead to preferential inactivation of the normal X chromosome to preserve the autosomal gene expression because the genetic information from the autosomal chromosome is deemed more essential and allowed to remain active. To learn more about the relationship between pigmentary mosaicisms and the genes involved in pigmentation, these investigators created a database of cytogenetic abnormalities reported in cases of pigmentary mosaicism (including reported cases of HI and LWNH). They noted that cytogenetic abnormalities overlapping with one or more genes involved in pigmentation were found in 88% of cases.[2] Abnormalities in karyotype can be detected in 30% to 60% of patients with HI or LWNH.[2] However, this relatively high percentage likely represents a reporting bias, because cases that have no karyotype abnormality may be underreported.

SEGMENTAL PIGMENTARY DISORDER
Hypopigmentation

Hypopigmented areas of SegPD are also commonly named *nevoid hypomelanosis* or *segmental nevus depigmentosus*. Localized hypopigmentation must be differentiated from ash leaf macules and confetti hypopigmentation associated with tuberous sclerosis (TS). Hypopigmented patches seen in TS are often smooth-bordered and oval-shaped (ash leaf macules) or small individual macules that do not follow a blaschkoid pattern. Hypopigmentation SegPD with hypopigmentation can also be differentiated from disorders such as vitiligo, which lead to depigmented areas that appear more starkly white and highlight distinctly with a Wood's lamp examination.

Hyperpigmentation

SegPD that is hyperpigmented is often called *nevoid hypermelanosis* or *segmental café au lait*. Large areas of hyperpigmented can be associated with McCune-Albright syndrome (polyostotic fibrous dysplasia with endocrinopathies such as precocious puberty). Large isolated café au lait macules associated with segmental neurofibromatosis tend to be more of a large oval or rectangular shape instead of the wavy and streaky blaschkoid pigmentation of nevoid hypermelanosis (see **Fig. 2**).

SYNDROMES ASSOCIATED WITH PATTERNED PIGMENTATION
Hypomelanosis of Ito

HI is characterized by linear and whorled hypopigmented streaks in the skin. HI is most commonly associated with neurologic abnormalities, such as seizures, delayed neurologic development, and macrocephaly, and abnormalities in the ocular, cardiac, and musculoskeletal systems are described in some cases. Currently many experts feel that the diagnosis of HI should be reserved for individuals who have the characteristic patterned hypopigmentation and neurologic abnormalities, and should not be given to those who only have the skin manifestations. However, earlier case reports do not always distinguish between these groups.

HI was originally described as *incontinentia pigmenti achromians* because the final stage of incontinentia pigmenti (IP) resembles the streaky hypopigmentation of HI, but HI lacks the preceding vesicular and verrucous stages (described later).[11] The term *IP achromians* should be abandoned because it can be confused with true IP.

The streaks in HI are typically present at birth but may be difficult to notice in very–fair-skinned children until their skin melanizes. HI does not represent a single genetic/chromosomal disorder, but is a cutaneous phenotype and has been associated with many different genetic abnormalities, including chromosomal translocations, insertions, aneuploidy, and microdeletions, often leading to chromosomal mosaicism.[2,10,12–14] A genetic abnormality is not always found.

The variability in the clinical presentation is likely from the large number of distinct genetic abnormalities that can lead to the same clinical phenotype of streaky hypopigmentation. Although neurologic abnormalities such as seizures, developmental delay, and macrocephaly are most common, the list of associated underlying abnormalities, including musculoskeletal, cardiac, and ophthalmologic, is long. Some of the more common associations are summarized in **Table 1**.[15–17] Approximately 30% to 90% of children (depending on the study) may have extracutaneous manifestations[15–17]; however, this is likely an overestimate because children who only have skin changes may never seek medical attention and are often not reported. It is also likely that the more widespread the skin pigmentary anomaly is the more likely systemic manifestations are present, perhaps because more of the ectodermal cells have the genetic defect. Although the number of associations can seem overwhelming, this is likely because of the large variability in genetic abnormalities, and therefore any one child is unlikely to have all of the manifestations described.

LINEAR AND WHORLED NEVOID HYPERMELANOSIS

LWNH is a disorder very similar to HI but with hyperpigmented streaks instead of hypopigmentation (**Fig. 3**). *LWNH* is preferred over the term *progressive cribiform and zosteriform hyperpigmentation* because the pigmentation does not follow

Table 1
Abnormalities commonly associated with hypomelanosis of Ito

Systemic Associations with HI	Organ System
Central nervous system	Neurodevelopmental delay
	Seizures
	Microcephaly
	Hydrocephalus
	Hypotonia
Musculoskeletal	Syndactyly, polydactyly, clinodactyly
	Short stature
	Scoliosis
	Coarse faces
Ophthalmologic	Congenital cataract
Cardiac	Congenital heart disease (VSD, PDA, tetralogy of Fallot)
Dental	Second molar agenesis, enamel defects
Other	Choanal atresia
	Impaired hearing
	Inguinal hernia

Abbreviations: HI, hypomelanosis of Ito; PDA, patent ductus artery; VSD, ventricular septal defect.
Data from Refs.[15–17]

dermatomes but instead lines of Blaschko, and is also preferred over the older terms *zebra-like pigmentation*, *zebra-like hyperpigmentation in whorls and streaks*, and *reticulate hyperpigmentation of Iijima*.[18,19] LWNH must again be differentiated from incontinentia pigmenti, which presents with vesicles, bullae, and verrucous plaques that eventually resolve with hyperpigmentation.

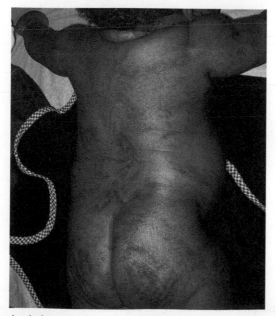

Fig. 3. Linear and whorled nevoid hypermelanosis in an infant.

LWNH has been reported to be associated with a similar constellation of neurologic, developmental, musculoskeletal, and, rarely, cardiac abnormalities to HI, but less frequently according to the two largest case series.[17,20] Di Lernia[20] noted that none of the 16 patients in their series who had unilateral hyperpigmentation had associated findings. This finding highlights the concept that localized dyspigmentation may be less likely associated with extracutaneous anomalies.

INCONTINENTIA PIGMENTI

IP (Bloch-Sulzberger disease) is neurocutaneous disorder characterized by a neonatal onset of skin lesions following the lines of Blaschko that show vesicular, verrucous, hyperpigmented, and, finally, hypopigmented stages (**Fig. 4**). IP is often associated with seizures or neurodevelopmental delay, ophthalmologic findings, absent or conical-shaped teeth, alopecia, and occasional cardiologic abnormalities. When present, seizures typically arise in the first few months of life but only occur in 13% of affected individuals.[21] Women who have very mild disease may show very limited signs as adults, including missing teeth, alopecia, and a localized area of linear hypo-pigmentation, and the skin eruption that was present in childhood may have been forgotten. Therefore, a careful maternal history, including input from the infant's maternal grandparent, may prove helpful if IP is suspected. Unlike HI, IP is a unique disorder caused by an X-linked dominant defect in the nuclear factor-κβ essential modulator (NEMO) pathway affecting nuclear factor-κβ. This transcription factor is critical to many immune and inflammatory pathways. IP is lethal in XY men because they cannot inactivate the abnormal X chromosome unless the mutation is localized to a small area, such as an arm or leg. Men with XXY karyotype may also survive if

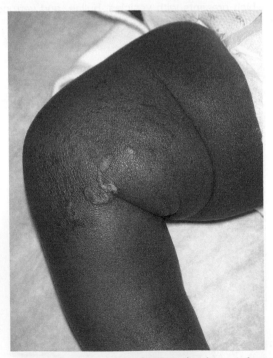

Fig. 4. Verrucous plaques and streaky hyperpigmentation in an infant with incontinentia pigmenti.

one X chromosome is unaffected. Because IP is one disorder instead of a group of genotypically distinct entities (as seen in HI and LWNH), the list of associated anomalies is less varied and genetic testing is available.

SYSTEMATIZED EPIDERMAL NEVUS

A verrucous epidermal nevus is a benign outgrowth of the top layer of the skin that can be either localized or "systematized." Localized lesions are very common, and present with an area of brown pigmentation typically in a line of Blaschko, which may start verrucous or flat in childhood and then become more verrucous. The terms *systematized epidermal nevus* or *epidermal nevus syndrome* are reserved for widespread involvement with either verrucous epidermal nevi or combined lesions with features of nevus sebaceus. This neurocutaneous disorder may be associated with underlying neurologic, ophthalmologic, or musculoskeletal anomalies. These disorders will be discussed in detail in article on epidermal nevi by Morel and Brandling Bennett elsewhere in this issue. Because epidermal nevi follow lines of Blaschko, are often hyperpigmented, and can be very flat in childhood, they may be difficult to differentiate from LWNH in infancy. A skin biopsy can often distinguish these, if necessary.

Table 2 summarizes selected skin disorders that also arise in the lines of Blaschko but have other distinctive features.

EVALUATION OF PATTERNED PIGMENTATION

SegPD is infrequently associated with an underlying systemic anomaly, and therefore workup should be guided by specific signs or symptoms.[4] Patients with widespread patterned pigmentation, especially those presenting with streaky, thin, Blaschkoid pigmentation, warrant a workup.

The initial workup of a patient with widespread streaky hypopigmentation or hyperpigmentation includes a thorough history, including a birth and family history of any pigmentary, skin, hair, or teeth anomalies to identify children with IP, and a thorough physical examination. If the pigmentation anomaly is widespread and the child is presenting in infancy, referral to neurology for a thorough baseline examination to evaluate for any subtle delays or motor defects would be reasonable, as would a baseline ophthalmologic examination. Genetic evaluation (including karyotype testing) is also important in children with extensive patterned pigmentation or if other organ systems are associated with the pigment changes.

Table 2	
Selected skin disorders arising in the lines of Blaschko	
Syndrome/Disease	**Skin Manifestations**
Congenital hemidysplasia with icthyosiform erythroderma and limb defects (CHILD syndrome)	Unilateral icthyosiform erythroderma
X-linked dominant chondrodysplasia punctata (Conradi-Hünermann syndrome)	Icthyosiform erythroderma in Blaschko's lines
Focal dermal hypoplasia (Goltz syndrome)	Fat herniations and linear atrophic streaks in Blaschko's lines
Lichen striatus	Thin blaschkoid lines of papules that flatten to become hypopigmented and resolve within 18 months

SUMMARY

The terms *pigmentary mosaicism* or *patterned dyspigmentation* describe a spectrum of clinical findings that range from localized areas of dyspigmentation with no systemic findings to widespread dyspigmentation with associated neurologic, musculoskeletal, and cardiac abnormalities, and other sequelae that can rarely lead to early demise. Given this wide spectrum, these patients must be approached with caution, but with the understanding that most who have localized pigmentary anomalies (SegPD) seem to have no systemic manifestations. These patients can be approached in many different ways, but generally children with more widespread dyspigmentation, and any with associated abnormalities or not meeting neurodevelopmental milestones, should be evaluated closely. Children with any red flags warrant subspecialty referral, and all children deserve close clinical follow-up with their primary care physician to ensure they meet all of their developmental milestones. Fortunately, parents can be reassured that most children with SegPD, and many with more widespread patterned pigmentation, are otherwise healthy.

REFERENCES

1. Happle R. Mosaicism in human skin. Understanding the patterns and mechanisms. Arch Dermatol 1993;129(11):1460–70.
2. Taibjee SM, Bennett DC, Moss C. Abnormal pigmentation in hypomelanosis of Ito and pigmentary mosaicism: the role of pigmentary genes. Br J Dermatol 2004; 151(2):269–82.
3. Lombillo VA, Sybert VP. Mosaicism in cutaneous pigmentation. Curr Opin Pediatr 2005;17(4):494–500.
4. Hogeling M, Frieden IJ. Segmental pigmentation disorder. Br J Dermatol 2010; 162(6):1337–41.
5. Metzker A, Morag C, Weitz R. Segmental pigmentation disorder. Acta Derm Venereol 1983;63:167–9.
6. Paller AS. Pigmentary patterning as a clinical clue of genetic mosaicism. Arch Dermatol 1996;132(10):1234–5.
7. Lyon MF. Sex chromatin and gene action in the mammalian X-chromosome. Am J Hum Genet 1962;14:135–48.
8. Happle R. Lyonization and the lines of Blaschko. Hum Genet 1985;70(3):200–6.
9. Happle R. Tentative assignment of hypomelanosis of Ito to 9q33–qter. Hum Genet 1987;75(1):98–9.
10. Koiffmann CP, de Souza DH, Diament A, et al. Incontinentia pigmenti achromians (hypomelanosis of ITO, MIM 146150): further evidence of localization at Xp11. Am J Med Genet 1993;46(5):529–33.
11. Ito M. Studies on melanin. Tohoku J Exp Med 1952;55(Suppl 1):1–104.
12. Ritter CL, Steele MW, Wenger SL, et al. Chromosome mosaicism in hypomelanosis of Ito. Am J Med Genet 1990;35(1):14–7.
13. Pellegrino JE, Schnur RE, Kline R, et al. Mosaic loss of 15q11q13 in a patient with hypomelanosis of Ito: is there a role for the P gene? Hum Genet 1995;96(4): 485–9.
14. Lungarotti MS, Martello C, Calabro A, et al. Hypomelanosis of Ito associated with chromosomal translocation involving Xp11. Am J Med Genet 1991;40(4): 447–8.
15. Ruiz-Maldonado R, Toussaint S, Tamayo L, et al. Hypomelanosis of Ito: diagnostic criteria and report of 41 cases. Pediatr Dermatol 1992;9(1):1–10.

16. Gomez-Lado C, Eiris-Punal J, Blanco-Barca O, et al. Hypomelanosis of Ito. A possibly under-diagnosed heterogeneous neurocutaneous syndrome. Rev Neurol 2004;38(3):223–8 [in Spanish].
17. Nehal KS, PeBenito R, Orlow SJ. Analysis of 54 cases of hypopigmentation and hyperpigmentation along the lines of Blaschko. Arch Dermatol 1996;132(10): 1167–70.
18. Rower JM, Carr RD, Lowney ED. Progressive cribiform and zosteriform hyperpigmentation. Arch Dermatol 1978;114(1):98–9.
19. Di Lernia V, Patrizi A, Neri I, et al. Reticulate hyperpigmentation of Iijima, Naito and Uyeno and other linear hyperpigmentations of children. Acta Derm Venereol 1992;72(5):393.
20. Di Lernia V. Linear and whorled hypermelanosis. Pediatr Dermatol 2007;24(3): 205–10.
21. Carney RG. Incontinentia pigmenti: a world statistical analysis. Arch Dermatol 1976;112:535–42.

The Diagnostic and Clinical Significance of Café-au-lait Macules

Kara N. Shah, MD, PhD[a,b],*

KEYWORDS

- Café-au-lait • Neurofibromatosis • NF-1

DEFINITION

Café-au-lait, also referred to as café-au-lait spots or café-au-lait macules, present as well-circumscribed, evenly pigmented macules and patches that range in size from 1 to 2 mm to greater than 20 cm in greatest diameter (**Fig. 1**). In light-skinned persons, the color appears light brown, or "coffee with milk," whereas in darker-skinned patients the color may appear as a medium to dark brown hue. Morphologically, café-au-lait have often been described as appearing either oval and smooth-bordered, resembling the "coast of California," or with jagged contours resembling the "coast of Maine." Although it has been suggested that the smooth-bordered, "coast of California" café-au-lait are more typical of the café-au-lait seen in neurofibro-matosis type 1 (NF-1) whereas those with the more jagged "coast of California" are more indicative of the café-au-lait seen in McCune-Albright syndrome, in clinical practice there appears to be a wide variability in morphology, such that this generalization is not diagnostically significant. Isolated, large café-au-lait may be seen on the torso or extremities (**Fig. 2**).

Histologically, café-au-lait demonstrate an increase in melanin content of both melanocytes and basal keratinocytes.[1] Giant melanosomes (macromelanosomes) may be seen. Both an increase in the number of melanocytes and an increase in the concentration of melanin and macromelanosomes has been reported in the

Disclosure: The author has nothing to disclose.

a Department of Pediatrics and Dermatology, University of Pennsylvania School of Medicine, Philadelphia, PA 19104, USA

b Division of General Pediatrics, The Children's Hospital of Philadelphia, 3550 Market Street, Room 2040, Philadelphia, PA 19104, USA

* Division of General Pediatrics, The Children's Hospital of Philadelphia, 3550 Market Street, Room 2040, Philadelphia, PA 19104.

E-mail address: shahk@email.chop.edu

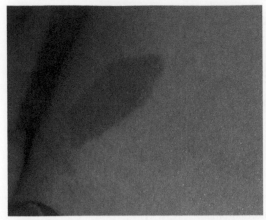

Fig. 1. Café-au-lait. Characteristic features include even pigmentation and smooth, well-defined borders.

café-au-lait associated with NF-1 as opposed to sporadic café-au-lait.[2,3] Proliferation of melanocytes is not seen.

EPIDEMIOLOGY AND NATURAL HISTORY

Solitary café-au-lait are common birthmarks. The presence of more than one café-au-lait, however, is less common. The frequency of multiple lesions, which has significance regarding the requirement for additional evaluation, has been examined in several population-based studies. Overall, the presence of one or more café-au-lait appears more common in African Americans than in Caucasians. The overall prevalence of at least one café-au-lait was noted to be present in 2.5% of neonates among 18,155 newborns of Caucasian, African American, Latino, and mixed-race ethnicity.[4] In this same study, one café-au-lait was noted in 0.3% of Caucasian newborns and 12% of African American newborns; 3 or more café-au-lait were seen in 1.8% of African American newborns but not in any Caucasian newborns. In a heterogeneous population of 4641 neonates in Boston, the overall prevalence of café-au-lait was noted to be 2.7% with at least one café-au-lait noted in 0.3% of Caucasian newborns and 18.3% of black newborns; none of the Caucasian infants was noted to have more than one café-au-lait, although in black infants 4.4% were noted to have 2 and 1.8%

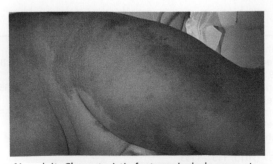

Fig. 2. Segmental café-au-lait. Characteristic features include even pigmentation with well-demarcated but "ragged" borders.

had 3 or more café-au-lait.[5] In infants and preschool-aged children, the prevalence of at least one café-au-lait increases to 25% of children as determined from a Baltimore cohort of 365 children aged 1 month through 5 years.[6] Whereas one café-au-lait was noted in 18.9% of children, the presence of 3 or more café-au-lait were seen in only 1.1% of children, and overall only 0.7% of otherwise normal children had 2 or more café-au-lait. In school-aged children, at least one café-au-lait has been noted in 22% to 36% of children.[7-10] Overall, the presence of 2 café-au-lait was reported to occur in 4.1% of a cohort of 732 Caucasian children from Nottingham, United Kingdom, and 3 café-au-lait were reported to occur in only 1.2% of children; the presence of 5 or more café-au-lait were seen in only 0.7% of children, and 60% of these children, all of whom had 6 or more café-au-lait, were presumed to have NF-1.[6] In a population of 1123 white Australian children aged 6 to 15 years, 26.1% were noted to have one café-au-lait, 6.9% to have 2 café-au-lait, and 3.3% to have 3 or more café-au-lait.[9]

Although many café-au-lait are present at birth, they may also manifest within the first few years of life. In fair-skinned infants they may be difficult to perceive on routine physical examination, but may be accentuated with examination under a Wood lamp. In general, it is unusual for additional sporadic café-au-lait to develop after the age of 6 years; in syndromes such as NF-1, however, new café-au-lait may continue to develop throughout childhood and adulthood. Sporadic café-au-lait often have been noted to fade in adulthood, whereas those associated with syndromes such as NF-1 do not.[11] Café-au-lait may develop anywhere on the body, although they more commonly occur on the torso, buttocks, and lower extremities and are uncommon on the face. During childhood they increase in size proportionate to the growth of the child. There does not appear to be any significant risk of malignant melanoma arising in a café-au-lait; only 2 case reports have been presented in the literature and likely occurred in combination by chance alone.[12,13]

PATHOGENESIS

Although café-au-lait may be seen anywhere on the body, they appear to be most common on the torso and occur rarely on the face, suggesting that sunlight exposure is not involved in the pathogenesis. An increase in the secretion of hepatocyte growth factor (HGF) and stem cell factor (SCF) by dermal fibroblasts has been reported in café-au-lait associated with NF-1, suggesting that these growth factors may be associated with the increased epidermal melanization observed in at least some café-au-lait.

DIFFERENTIAL DIAGNOSIS

Although café-au-lait are usually readily diagnosed on examination, occasionally they may be difficult to differentiate from other pigmented lesions (Table 1). At times, café-au-lait may be difficult to distinguish from other pigmented birthmarks, including congenital melanocytic nevi, speckled lentiginous nevus, Becker nevus, and forms of pigmentary mosaicism such as nevoid hypermelanosisand segmental pigmentation disorder. Acquired pigmentary lesions, including ephelides (freckles), lentigo, and postinflammatory hyperpigmentation may also be mistaken for café-au-lait. The lesions of urticaria pigmentosa or solitary mastocytomas, which are benign manifestations of cutaneous mastocytosis, are often mistaken for café-au-lait as they are usually noted during infancy as acquired, light-brown macules scattered on the torso, buttocks, and extremities. They may be easily distinguished in most children by eliciting Darier's sign, or the development of urticaria with firm stroking, which triggers mast cell degranulation. Blistering may sometimes occur, most commonly during infancy.

Table 1
Differential diagnosis of café-au-lait

Diagnosis	Clinical Features
Ephelides	"Freckles"; 1–2-mm light brown macules on sun-exposed areas; darken with sun exposure and fade in winter
Lentigenes	Darkly pigmented, well-circumscribed 1–2-mm macules; usually solitary but may be more numerous; commonly associated with sun exposure
Congenital melanocytic nevus	Light-brown to dark-brown, usually well-circumscribed macules, patches or plaques; may be associated with hypertrichosis; although many are uniform in color, areas of darker pigmentation may be noted
Becker nevus	Acquired light brown patch that usually develops during adolescence; more common in males; usually seen on the shoulder upper chest or upper back; associated with hypertrichosis
Pigmentary mosaicism	Irregular, light-brown to medium-brown patches, often with jagged borders, that typically present at birth or in early infancy; may be referred to as nevoid hypermelanosis. Larger patches, referred to as segmental pigmentary disorder, may be seen on the torso and demonstrate a well-defined midline border and less well-defined lateral border represent a form of cutaneous mosaicism
Postinflammatory hyperpigmentation	Poorly defined hyperpigmented macules and patches that develop at sites of prior trauma or inflammation; there may be associated atrophic or hypertrophic scarring; usually fade over time
Speckled lentiginous nevus	Congenital light-brown patch that develops acquired pigmented lesions within, usually junctional or compound melanocytic nevi
Urticaria pigmentosa, mastocytoma	Light brown to medium brown, relatively well-circumscribed congenital or acquired macules, papules, and plaques composed of increased numbers of cutaneous mast cells; often urticate when stroked or in response to heat, friction, or other exposures that trigger mast cell degranulation

EVALUATION

Presentation of a child with café-au-lait macules to the primary care provider, geneticist, or dermatologist is a common scenario. Two prospective cohort studies have attempted to define the predictive value of the number and morphology of café-au-lait macules in children with regard to eventual diagnosis of NF-1 or other disorders associated with café-au-lait. In one study, a cohort of 41 children with 6 or more café-au-lait greater than 5 mm in diameter was followed prospectively.[14] The children ranged in age from 1 month to 10 years at initial evaluation and were followed clinically over a period of at least 2 years. Fifty-eight percent of children were eventually diagnosed with NF-1 using established clinical criteria, predominantly based on the presence of axillary and/or inguinal freckling, with Lisch nodules and cutaneous neurofibromas developing in only a few patients each. The mean age at diagnosis of skin-fold freckling was 4.4 years, with a range of 18 months to 11.6 years. Lisch nodules were noted at a mean age of 3.7 years, with a range of 1.2 to 7.5 years. Six children were noted to have features of segmental neurofibromatosis with café-au-lait and skin-fold freckling only without other manifestations of NF-1. When those patients who were diagnosed with segmental neurofibromatosis or another disorder were excluded, NF-1 was diagnosed in 75% of children. Seventy-five percent of children were diagnosed with NF-1 on the basis of consensus criteria by 6 years of age, and the majority by 10 years. Of note, 8 children were diagnosed with multiple café-au-lait only without any other stigmata of NF-1; one of these children was also noted to have severe developmental delay but no other unifying diagnosis. One patient each was diagnosed with Banayan-Riley-Ruvalcaba syndrome, LEOPARD/multiple lentigenes syndrome, and McCune-Albright/polyostotic fibrous dysplasia, respectively. In a smaller cohort of 21 patients with 6 or more café-au-lait 5 mm or larger, 8 of 14 children with "typical" café-au-lait were diagnosed with NF-1; in the remaining 6 patients with NF-1, the diagnosis was suspected on the basis of nondiagnostic clinical features but was unconfirmed. Only 1 patient of 5 with "atypical" café-au-lait was suspected of having NF-1.[15]

More recently, a cohort of 110 children aged 1 to 206 months referred for evaluation to a single NF-1 center on the basis of the presence of one or more café-au-lait was followed for a period of 4 years.[16] Thirty-one percent of children met clinical criteria for NF-1 during the study period. Of the children with 6 or more café-au-lait at presentation, 77% were eventually diagnosed with NF-1. No child with less than 6 café-au-lait was diagnosed with NF-1. The children eventually diagnosed with NF-1 had a mean of 11.8 café-au-lait (ranging from 6 to more than 20). In patients with "typical" café-au-lait (those with even pigmentation and smooth, distinct borders, usually round or oval in shape), 32 of 68 (47%) eventually met criteria for NF-1 compared with 2 of 42 (4.7%) of those patients with "atypical" café-au-lait (those with irregular or smudgy borders or nonhomogeneous pigmentation), both of whom had greater than 6 café-au-lait. The mean age at diagnosis of NF-1 was 33.5 months; 76% met criteria for diagnosis by 4 years of age, 94% met criteria for diagnosis at 6 years of age, and all were diagnosed by 8 years of age. The most common diagnostic feature in addition to café-au-lait was axillary or inguinal freckling, which was observed in 77% of patients.

CLINICAL PRESENTATIONS

Although neurofibromatosis-1 is the most common and well-recognized syndrome associated with café-au-lait, they have been associated with several other syndromes, including neurofibromatosis-2 (NF-2), McCune-Albright syndrome, and Noonan syndrome. A review of the features of many of the syndromes associated with café-au-lait is presented in **Table 2**. Although comprehensive, this list is not exhaustive, and for many of these syndromes the evidence that café-au-lait occur with more frequency than in the general population is weak because overall, the presence of 1 to 2 café-au-lait is relatively common.

Neurofibromatosis Type 1

Although von Recklinghausen is generally credited with the earliest systematic description of the clinical features of neurofibromatosis-1, which was previously known as von Recklinghausen disease, café-au-lait macules were not initially recognized as a prominent feature of this disease. Crowe published the first association of café-au-lait with neurofibromatosis in the English literature, and although the cohort of 98 institutionalized patients he described likely was composed not only of patients with what we now recognize as NF-1 but also with patients with other forms of neurofibromatosis, including familial spinal neurofibromatosis and segmental neurofibromatosis, he noted that "not a single adult was found with 6 or more café-au-lait spots who

Table 2
Syndromes associated with café-au-lait macules

Strength of Association	Syndrome	Clinical Features	Gene or Locus
Strong	Neurofibromatosis type 1	Multiple café-au-lait, skin-fold freckling, Lisch nodules, optic pathway glioma, skeletal dysplasia, cutaneous and plexiform neurofibromas, neurocognitive deficits, macrocephaly	NF-1
	Neurofibromatosis type 2	Acoustic neuromas, schwannomas, neurofibromas, meningiomas, juvenile posterior subcapsular lenticular opacity; café-au-lait seen but not a criterion for diagnosis	NF-2
	Multiple familial café-au-lait	Multiple café-au-lait without other stigmata of NF-1	?
	Legius (NF-1–like) syndrome	Multiple café-au-lait and skin-fold freckling without other stigmata of NF-1	SPRED1
	McCune-Albright syndrome	Segmental café-au-lait, precocious puberty, other endocrinopathies, polyostotic fibrous dysplasia	GNAS1
	Constitutional mismatch repair deficiency syndrome	Multiple café-au-lait, adenomatous colonic polyps, multiple malignancies, including colonic adenocarcinoma, glioblastoma, medulloblastoma, and lymphoma	MLH1, MSH2, MSH6, PMS2
	Ring chromosome syndromes	Multiple café-au-lait, microcephaly, mental retardation, short stature, skeletal anomalies	Chromosomes 7, 11, 12, 15, 17
	LEOPARD/multiple lentigenes syndrome	Café-au-lait, café-noir, lentigenes, cardiac conduction defects, ocular hypertelorism, pulmonary stenosis, genitourinary anomalies, growth retardation, hearing loss	PTPN11
	Cowden syndrome (multiple hamartoma syndrome)	Facial trichilemmomas, cobblestoning of the oral mucosa, predisposition to soft tissue tumors (lipomas, neuromas), gastrointestinal polyps, fibrocystic breast disease and breast carcinoma, thyroid adenoma and thyroid cancer	PTEN
	Banayan-Riley-Ruvalcalba syndrome	Facial trichilemmomas, oral papillomas, pigmented genital macules, gastrointestinal polyps, macrocephaly, vascular anomalies, mental retardation	PTEN
Weak	Ataxia-telangiectasia	Cerebellar ataxia, cutaneous and ocular telangiectasias, immunodeficiency, hypogonadism, predisposition to lymphoreticular malignancy	ATM
	Bloom syndrome	Photosensitivity, immunodeficiency, chronic lung disease, cryptorchidism, syndactyly, short stature, susceptibility to malignancy	RECQL3

Syndrome	Features	Gene/Locus
Fanconi anemia	Bone marrow failure, multiple congenital anomalies, predisposition to malignancy, mental retardation, microcephaly	FANCA, FANCB (putative), FANCC, FANCD locus on chromosome 3, FANCE locus on chromosome 6, FANCF, FANCG, FANCH (putative)
Russell-Silver syndrome	Short stature, craniofacial and body asymmetry, low birth weight, microcephaly, triangular facies, fifth finger clinodactyly, congenital cardiac defects	?
Tuberous sclerosis	Facial angiofibromas, cutaneous collagenomas, seizures, mental retardation, hypomelanotic macules, periungual fibromas, subependymal nodules, subependymal giant cell astrocytoma, cardiac rhabdomyoma, pulmonary lymphangiomyomatosis renal angiomyolipoma, retinal hamartomas	TSC1, TSC2
Turner syndrome	Short stature, lymphedema, congenital heart disease, valgus deformity	X-chromosomal anomalies (XO karyotype or Xp deletion)
Noonan syndrome	Facial dysmorphism, pulmonary valve stenosis, webbed neck, pectus excavatum, mental retardation, short stature, cryptorchidism, hematologic malignancies	PTPN11, SOS1, RAF1, KRAS
Multiple mucosal neuroma (MEN) syndrome 1	Parathyroid adenoma, pituitary adenoma, pancreatic islet adenoma, lipoma, gingival papules, facial angiofibromas, collagenomas	MENIN
MEN syndrome 2B	Mucosal neuromas, pheochromocytoma, medullary thyroid carcinoma, parathyroid adenoma, marfanoid habitus	RET
Johanson-Blizzard syndrome	Short stature, failure to thrive, microcephaly, sensorineural hearing loss, dental anomalies, congenital heart disease, exocrine pancreatic insufficiency, imperforate anus, genitourinary anomalies, mental retardation, hypothyroidism	UBR1
Microcephalic osteodysplastic primordial dwarfism, type II	Short stature, microcephaly, intrauterine growth retardation, dysmorphic facies, skeletal anomalies, developmental delay, premature puberty	PCNT2
Nijmegen breakage syndrome	Short stature, growth retardation, microcephaly, cleft lip/palate, dysmorphic facies, bronchiectasis, sinusitis, dysgammaglobulinemia with recurrent urinary tract and gastrointestinal infections, mental retardation, spontaneous chromosomal instability, predisposition to malignancy	NBS1
Rubinstein-Taybi syndrome	Short stature, microcephaly, dysmorphic facies, congenital cardiac disease, sternal anomalies, skeletal anomalies, mental retardation	CREBBP, EP300
Kabuki syndrome	Postnatal growth retardation, microcephaly, dysmorphic facies, congenital cardiac defects, malabsorption, anal stenosis, genitourinary anomalies, congenital hip dysplasia, hirsutism, mental retardation	?

did not also have neurofibromata" and "the fewer the number of café-au-lait spots the more marked was the central involvement, as characterized by central nervous system, intrathoracic, or retroperitoneal tumors."[17] Of note, in Crowe's original study of neurofibromatosis patients (likely representing a mixed population of patients with NF-1, NF-2, schwannomatosis, and segmental neurofibromatosis), 22% had less than 6 café-au-lait and 5% had none.

The majority of children with NF-1 have multiple café-au-lait scattered predominantly on the torso, buttocks, and legs, although they may occur anywhere (**Fig. 3**). The macules are classically described as having a smooth, "coast of California" border, although it is well known that café-au-lait with a less typical morphology also occur in NF-1. Café-au-lait are usually the first presenting sign of NF-1, although in young children they may be overlooked or, in fair-skinned infants, difficult to appreciate on physical examination. The spots are often present at birth, and frequently increase in number during the first 6 to 10 years of life; they increase in size proportionate to the growth of the child and darken with sun exposure. There is no association between number of café-au-lait and severity of NF-1.

Diagnostic criteria for NF-1 were established in 1988 by a National Institutes of Health Consensus Conference and revised in 1997.[18,19] The presence of 2 or more of the following criteria is required to establish the diagnosis.

- Six or more café-au-lait ≥5 mm in prepubertal individual or ≥15 mm in a postpubertal individual
- Two or more neurofibromas of any type or one plexiform neurofibroma
- Axillary and/or inguinal freckling
- Optic pathway glioma
- Two or more Lisch nodules
- A distinctive osseous lesion, including sphenoid wing dysplasia or thinning of the long bone cortex with or without pseudarthrosis
- A first-degree relative (parent, sibling, offspring) with confirmed NF-1.

Lisch nodules are benign, asymptomatic iris hamartomas that are pathognomonic for NF-1. These nodules are typically only visualized under slit-lamp examination and usually develop during childhood. Optic pathway gliomas (OPG) are present in about 15% of patients with NF-1, but are considered indolent tumors with a low incidence of progression to symptomatic presentation, with only about 30% becoming symptomatic. These gliomas may be noted on fundoscopic examination, incidentally

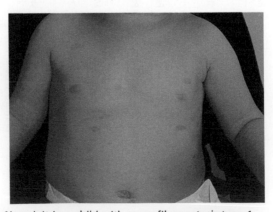

Fig. 3. Multiple café-au-lait in a child with neurofibromatosis type 1.

on radiologic examination, or may present with proptosis, decreased visual acuity, visual field defects, headache, or precocious puberty; most are diagnosed by 3 years of age.[20,21] Current recommendations for screening for OPG in children with NF-1 do not include the routine use of magnetic resonance imaging but do include annual full ophthalmologic evaluation through age 6 years with less frequent evaluation after age 6 years.[20,21] Sphenoid wing dysplasia and cortical thinning and dysplasia of the long bones are peculiar osseous malformations seen in NF-1 that represent congenital mesodermal dysplasias. Sphenoid wing dysplasia may be noted on careful physical examination or on radiologic imaging of the facial bones. Cortical thinning and dysplasia of the long bones are usually congenital in origin and may present with anterolateral bowing of the tibia and subsequent pathologic fractures during the first year of life with resultant pseudoarthoses; any long bone may be involved, but the tibia, humerus, and femur are the most commonly affected sites.

Use of the diagnostic criteria for NF-1 has been validated in the diagnosis of NF-1 in children. In a large cohort of 1402 patients younger than 21 years who were diagnosed with NF-1 after evaluation at a neurofibromatosis clinic, 97% met 2 or more criteria by 8 years of age, and all met criteria by 20 years of age.[22] However, 30% of infants diagnosed with NF-1 before 1 year of age presented with only one criterion in addition to an affected first-degree relative, and overall 46% of sporadic cases did not meet criteria at 1 year of age, suggesting that diagnosis in infants for whom there is no family history is difficult if they are younger than 1 year. Ninety-nine percent of NF-1 patients presented with 6 of more café-au-lait 5 mm or larger by 1 year of age. Inguinal and/or axillary freckling was noted in 90% of patients by 7 years of age, and Lisch nodules were seen on slit-lamp examination in more than 70% of affected children by 10 years of age. In contrast, neurofibromas were seen in only 48% of children by 10 years of age and 84% of patients by 20 years of age. Osseous lesions are usually noted within the first year of life and were noted in 14% of patients. Symptomatic optic pathway glioma was noted in 1% of patients by 1 year of age and in 4% by 3 years of age. Excellent reviews of the clinical features of NF-1, including both the cutaneous and extracutaneous manifestations, have been published recently.[23–25]

Skin-fold freckling, also known as Crowe's sign, presents as multiple 1- to 3-mm pigmented macules resembling small café-au-lait and is reportedly the most specific of the NF-1 criteria; it is considered pathognomonic for NF-1[23] (**Fig. 4**). Skin-fold freckling often arises around 3 to 5 years of age, although it may be noted earlier and occasionally at birth.[26] In addition to the axillary and inguinal areas, skin-fold freckling may also involve the posterior neck, inframammary region, and perioral area.

Neurofibromas are benign nerve sheath tumors composed of Schwann cells, fibroblasts, mast cells, nerve axons, and perineural cells, and although not specific for NF-1, they are a cardinal feature. Neurofibromas are further characterized as cutaneous (dermal), subcutaneous, and plexiform. Cutaneous neurofibromas appear as rubbery, exophytic soft papules and nodules in the skin and may occur anywhere on the body. These lesions usually present during adolescence and increase in number during adulthood; they may eventually number in the hundreds.[27] Neurofibromas may cause significant disfigurement and pruritus. Cutaneous neurofibromas are not considered to have the potential for malignant degeneration. Subcutaneous neurofibromas appear as rubbery subcutaneous masses; they are often painful, and those that involve the dorsal root ganglia may cause symptoms of spinal cord compression. Malignant degeneration is uncommon. Plexiform neurofibromas are usually present at birth, although they may not become clinically apparent until later in childhood or in adulthood. Plexiform neurofibromas are clinically apparent in 27% of patients, although about 50% of adult NF-1 patients show evidence of plexiform

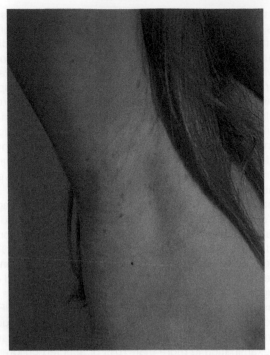

Fig. 4. Axillary freckling in a child with neurofibromatosis type 1.

neurofibromas on computed tomography imaging.[28] These lesions are typically large nodular tumors that develop along nerves. On examination, they feel like a "bag of worms." Associated overlying café-au-lait and/or hypertrichosis may be evident. Large, diffuse plexiform neurofibromas may cause significant pain, disfigurement, and compression of the skin, subcutis, and associated viscera. Plexiform neurofibromas are associated with the development of malignant peripheral nerve sheath tumors (MPNST), which are reported to occur in 8% to 12% of NF-1 patients.[29] Although plexiform neurofibromas are often noted to grow during childhood, the development of sudden, rapid growth, associated pain, or neurologic deficit should alert the clinician as to the possibility of malignant transformation. MPNST carry a poor prognosis; metastasis is common, and many are resistant to chemotherapy.

In addition to café-au-lait, skin-fold freckling, and cutaneous and plexiform neurofibromas, other cutaneous findings in NF-1 include generalized hyperpigmentation, blue-red macules, and pseudoatrophic macules; the latter 2 entities are believed to represent unusual variants of cutaneous neurofibromas. Juvenile xanthogranulomas, which are non-Langerhans cell histiocytic proliferations that most commonly involve the skin, have also been reported to occur more frequently in NF-1 than in the general population and to possibly indicate an increased risk of juvenile myelomonocytic leukemia, although these associations are questionable.[30,31] Other clinical features of NF-1 include relative macrocephaly (45%), short stature (30%), scoliosis (10%), pectus excavatum, cognitive deficits (including attention deficit hyperactivity disorder, learning disabilities, below average intelligence) (30%–60%), hypertension, vascular dysplasia, precocious puberty, and unidentified bright objects on brain magnetic resonance imaging.[32] Vascular dysplasia, including pulmonary stenosis, renal artery stenosis, and stenosis or occlusion of the internal carotid and cerebral arteries occurs in about 2% of children with NF-1.[33] In addition to MPNST, other malignancies reported to occur in association with NF-1 include pheochromocytoma, rhabdomyosarcomas, gastrointestinal stromal tumors, intracranial neoplasms, and juvenile myelomonocytic leukemia.[34–40] Neurofibromatous neuropathy is a symmetric, predominantly sensory polyneuropathy that may develop in NF-1 patients and is associated with the development of large numbers of cutaneous and subcutaneous neurofibromas.[41] Vitamin D deficiency, osteopenia, and osteoporosis have been reported to occur in adults and children with NF-1, and may be a predisposing factor in skeletal anomalies, including scoliosis.[42–44]

The prevalence of NF-1 is estimated to be between 1 in 2000 and 1 in 4500 persons.[45] NF-1 is an autosomal dominant disorder with 100% penetrance but broad variability in clinical manifestations.[46,47] The gene responsible for NF-1 was discovered in 1990, is localized on chromosome 17q11.2, and encodes the protein neurofibromin, a tumor suppressor involved in the intracellular Ras-guanosine triphosphate pathway, which regulates cell proliferation and differentiation.[48–50] Wild-type neurofibromin inhibits Ras-guanosine triphosphatase (GTPase) activity; when the NF1 gene is mutated, activation of Ras occurs and results in increased signaling through downstream effectors such as Raf and mitogen-activated protein kinase (MAPK).[51]

The NF1 gene has one of the highest spontaneous mutation rates among known human genes; approximately 50% of patients present with de novo mutations and therefore no family history of NF-1. Eighty to ninety percent of new mutations are paternally derived.[52,53] In addition, a wide variety of mutations have been described, including gene deletions, insertions, amino acid substitutions, chromosomal rearrangements, and splicing mutations.[54,55] There appears to be little genotype-phenotype correlation with the exception of patients with deletion of the entire NF1 gene as part of a contiguous gene deletion syndrome, which occurs in about 5% of all NF-1 patients; deletion of the entire NF1 gene is associated with a tendency to develop large number of neurofibromas, more severe cognitive deficits, and greater risk of developing MPNST.[56–59] Many of the known mutations in the NF1 gene are predicted to result in premature truncation of the neurofibromin protein. The NF1 gene is quite large, encompassing 60 exons and more than 300 kilobases of DNA; therefore detection of NF1 mutations is a difficult and time-consuming endeavor. A comprehensive mutation analysis of the NF1 gene now allows for identification of NF1 mutations in 95% of patients who meet clinical criteria for the diagnosis of NF-1.[60] Although penetrance appears to be nearly 100%, there is a significant degree of variability in expressivity, even among family members carrying the same NF1 mutation.[61] Genetic analysis of a panel of melanocyte-derived primary cell cultures from café-au-lait from 5 patients with NF-1 demonstrated not only the germline NF1 mutation but also a second mutation in the other NF1 gene.[62] Neurofibromas from patients with NF-1 have also been shown to possess not only the germline NF1 gene mutation but also a second-hit mutation in the NF1 gene.[63]

Segmental NF-1 is a variant of NF-1 that results from somatic mosaicism arising from postzygotic mutations in the NF1 gene, such that the clinical manifestations of NF-1 are present only in a localized body segment.[64–68] Mutations in NF1 have been demonstrated in café-au-lait and neurofibromas in these patients.[62,68] Bilateral presentations of segmental NF-1 have been reported.[69–74] Another variant of NF-1 is hereditary spinal neurofibromatosis, a rare disorder that generally presents with multiple café-au-lait and multiple, symmetric spinal root neurofibromas; skin-fold freckling may be present but other stigmata of NF-1 are typically absent.[75,76]

A subset of patients with NF-1 appears to manifest overlap in clinical features with Noonan syndrome, including pulmonary valve stenosis, "Noonan" facies, and pectus excavatum; these patients have been shown to manifest NF1 mutations.[77–80] Of note, both NF-1 and Noonan syndrome, in addition to several other genetic syndromes, display a remarkable overlap in clinical features, including pigmentary skin anomalies, facial dysmorphism, short stature, congenital heart defects, neurocognitive defects, and a predisposition to malignancy. Related disorders include Costello syndrome, cardiofaciocutaneous syndrome, and LEOPARD syndrome. These disorders have been collectively referred to as the neuro-cardio-facial-cutaneous syndromes, and they have all been shown to result from mutations in one or more of several genes involved in the Ras/Mitogen-activated protein kinase (RAS/MAPK) signaling pathway, which regulates cell proliferation and differentiation through several downstream effectors, including ERK (extracellular signal-regulated kinase).[51,81–83]

Familial Multiple Café-au-lait

Several reports have identified families in which multiple café-au-lait are present without any other stigmata of NF-1 and no evidence of mutation in the NF1 gene. Familial multiple café-au-lait appears to be transmitted as an autosomal dominant disorder; its relationship to NF-1 remains unclear and awaits further characterization at the genetic level.[84–87] This diagnosis should only be made in an older child when other features of NF-1 are absent and there is a clear family history of multiple café-au-lait without other stigmata of NF-1.

Legius Syndrome

The presence of familial café-au-lait in association with axillary and/or inguinal freck-ling but without the presence of Lisch nodules, neurofibromas, or other stigmata of NF-1 was recently demonstrated to be associated with mutations in the gene SPRED1 (Sprouty-related, EVH1 domain containing 1) in several families in whom no NF1 gene mutations were identified.[88] SPRED1 is a negative regulator of ERK, and SPRED1 specifically inhibits MAPK signaling by suppressing activation of Raf.[89] Previously known as NF-1–like syndrome, Legius syndrome is indistinguishable from NF-1 regarding number and pattern of distribution of café-au-lait and skin-fold freckling.[90] In the original cohort of 44 patients from 5 families, multiple café-au-lait were noted in each patient with a variable number manifesting skin-fold freckling, which was described as "mild"; other reported features included macrocephaly 97% or greater (29.5%), cutaneous lipomas (32%), Noonan-like facial dysmorphism (9%), attention-deficit/hyperactivity disorder (ADHD) and/or learning disability (9%), pectus excava-tum (7%) and supravalvular pulmonic stenosis (2%). No Lisch nodules, neurofibromas, OPG, or distinctive osseous lesions were noted.[88] A cohort of 42 patients with docu-mented SPRED1 mutations, including 23 probands and 19 relatives, were screened for the presence of café-au-lait, skin-fold freckling, and macrocephaly.[91] Twenty of these patients (47.6%) met clinical criteria for NF-1 based on 6 or more café-au-lait and skin-fold freckling. Skin-fold freckling, however, was reported as "mild or faint" in half of the affected patients. In addition, 34 of 1318 (2.6%) of patients from an anon-ymous cohort referred for NF1 genetic testing demonstrated a SPRED1 mutation. The majority of mutations were predicted to result in premature SPRED1 protein transla-tion. Overall, from the anonymous cohort, 1086 patients met clinical criteria for NF-1; 76% demonstrated an NF1 mutation, 1.9% demonstrated a SPRED1 mutation, and 22% failed to demonstrate either an NF1 or SPRED1 mutation. In the patients with documented SPRED1 mutations, there were no patients with Lisch nodules, neurofi-bromas, OPG, or the typical osseous lesions of NF-1. Several children with ADHD and/or abnormal language and speech development were noted.

Neurofibromatosis Type 2

In contrast to NF-1, NF-2 is significantly less common, with a prevalence of about 1:25,000 based on epidemiologic studies in England.[92] Penetrance approaches 100%.[92,93] Café-au-lait, although not a diagnostic criterion for NF-2, are present in 33% to 43% of patients; other cutaneous manifestations are seen in 59% to 68% of patients and include cutaneous schwannomas, which present as pigmented plaques and intradermal tumors, and cutaneous neurofibromas.[93–95] Although vestibular schwannomas, previously known as acoustic neuromas, are the most recognizable feature of this disorder, other diagnostic criteria include spinal schwannomas, neurofibromas, meningiomas, and gliomas.[92] The Manchester diagnostic criteria comprise the diagnostic standard for NF-2. Any one of the following sets of clinical manifestations is required for the diagnosis of NF-1[96]:

- Bilateral vestibular schwannomas
- First-degree relative with NF-2 plus unilateral vestibular schwannoma or two of meningioma, schwannoma, glioma, neurofibroma, or posterior subcapsular lenticular opacity
- Unilateral vestibular schwannoma plus two of meningioma, schwannoma, glioma, neurofibroma, or posterior subcapsular lenticular opacity
- Multiple meningiomas plus unilateral vestibular schwannoma or two of schwannoma, glioma, neurofibroma, posterior subcapsular lenticular opacity.

Schwannomas are benign, encapsulated tumors arising from the Schwann cells of cranial nerves 3 to 12, spinal nerves, and peripheral nerves; malignant degeneration is rare. The clinical and genetic features of NF-2 have recently been reviewed.[97] Although most patients present in early adulthood with hearing loss secondary to a vestibular schwannoma, often with associated tinnitus, dizziness, and vertigo, presentation during childhood may occur.[96,98] In children the most common presenting signs and symptoms include deafness, meningiomas, spinal schwannomas, cutaneous schwannomas, café-au-lait, early-onset lens opacities, visual abnormalities, and peripheral neuropathy.[99–101]

The gene for NF-2 is located on chromosome 22q11.2 and encompasses 17 coding exons. NF2 encodes the protein merlin (also known as schwannomin), which is believed to function as a tumor suppressor, and loss of merlin expression has been documented in NF-2–associated tumors.[102,103] There is a high rate of de novo mutations, with about 50% of patients lacking a family history of NF-2.[96] Somatic mosaicism has been reported with evidence for gonadal mosaicism and transmission of the mutated NF2 gene to offspring.[104] Genetic testing is available and can detect mutations in NF2 in 95% of patients who meet diagnostic criteria. Genotype-phenotype correlations exist.[105]

McCune-Albright Syndrome

McCune-Albright syndrome (MAS) is a rare, sporadic disorder; the incidence is unknown. The cardinal features include polyostotic fibrous dysplasia, precocious puberty and other endocrinopathies, and large, irregular segmental café-au-lait that typically involve the torso or buttocks. The differential diagnosis for the large café-au-lait that occurs in MAS includes segmental pigmentation disorder and segmental NF-1.[106–108] Diagnosis of MAS requires the presence of at least 2 of the 3 cardinal clinical features. Fibrous dysplasia is most commonly polyostotic, although monostotic presentation may be seen, and typically involves the long bones and base of the skull. Although these anomalies may be asymptomatic, pain, fracture and skeletal asymmetry may develop. Fibrous dysplasia has been reported in 46% to 98% of patients with MAS.[109,110] Severely affected persons may present at birth; although most children are diagnosed with MAS within the first few years of life with a mean age at diagnosis of 4.9 years. Precocious puberty is the most common presentation and is significantly more common in girls, which may account for the preponderance of this disorder in girls. MAS is frequently characterized by alternating progression and regression of pubertal development with atypical pubertal development. Precocious puberty has been reported in 64 to 94% of girls with MAS but in only 15% of boys.[110–113] Other endocrinologic abnormalities include hyperthyroidism, hyperparathyroidism, and acromegaly. Cardiac disease, hepatobiliary disease, nephrocalcinosis, renal phosphate wasting, and platelet dysfunction have also been reported in patients with MAS.[114–116]

The café-au-lait associated with MAS generally are large, unilateral, and often occur on the buttocks, chest, and posterior neck. Although clinically the café-au-lait of MAS are indistinguishable from those seen in NF-1, macromelanosomes are reportedly absent in the café-au-lait associated with MAS.[117] The café-au-lait seen in association with MAS are usually noted at birth or within the first few years of life, and are seen in 53% to 95% of patients with MAS.[109,112] Once present, they do not increase in number but do increase in size proportionate to the growth of the child. Accentuation with sun exposure occurs. The macules are commonly described as having a jagged, "coast of Maine" border, although this morphology is not uniformly present. The café-au-lait are distributed along the lines of Blaschko, which represent ectodermal migration patterns during embryogenesis and thus are a manifestation of the somatic mosaicism that underlies MAS.[118] Pigmentation of oral mucosa manifesting as melanotic macules has also been reported in MAS.[119,120]

MAS is caused by postzygotic mutations in the gene GNAS1, which encodes the α subunit of stimulatory G protein.[121,122] Only 4 missense mutations have been described in MAS; all of these mutations have been documented to involve arginine 201, which is critical for modulation of GTPase activity. Through their interaction with numerous G-protein–coupled receptors, G proteins regulate a variety of signal transduction pathways; in MAS, dysregulation of GTPase activity results in constitutive activation of adenylyl cyclase activity and increased intracellular cyclic adenosine monophosphate (AMP) levels.[123] Autonomous endocrine hyperfunction, increased melanogenesis, and dysregulation of cell proliferation all result from increased cyclic AMP–mediated intracellular signaling. Germline mutations in GNAS1 are proposed to be lethal, thus only embryos with somatic mutations survive; the resultant genetic mosaicism results in marked phenotypic variability.[124] Family history, therefore, is routinely negative. Within the skin, melanocytes derived from areas of café-au-lait have been shown to manifest activating mutations in GNAS1 with resultant increased cyclic AMP activity and increased tyrosinase activity.[125] Overall, however, genetic testing of skin from café-au-lait in patients with MAS for the presence of GNAS1 mutations yields an identifiable mutation in only 27% of affected patients, compared with 21% from peripheral blood, 82% from affected bone, and 100% from thyroid tissue as demonstrated in an analysis of 113 affected patients.[113] This finding has been attributed to the low proportion of melanocytes in affected skin, which renders detection of GNAS1 mutations difficult, even despite use of highly sensitive polymerase chain reaction–based analysis.

Constitutional Mismatch Repair Deficiency Syndrome

Recently, an association between the presence of multiple café-au-lait and skin-fold freckling without other stigmata of NF-1, adenomatous colonic polyps with early-onset colorectal carcinoma, and a predisposition to a variety of pediatric malignancies has emerged.[126] This syndrome has been variably termed constitutional mismatch repair deficiency (CMMR-D), Lynch III syndrome, and CoLoN (colon tumors and/or leukemia/lymphoma and/or neurofibromatosis features). Homozygous or compound heterozygous germline mutations in one of several genes involved in DNA mismatch repair have been identified in affected children, including MLH1, MSH2, MSH6, and PMS2. These genes have all been previously associated with hereditary nonpolyposis colorectal cancer, also referred to as Lynch syndrome.[127] The malignancies associated with CMMR-D include hematological malignancies, including non-Hodgkin lymphoma and acute lymphoblastic lymphoma; brain tumors, including glioblastoma multiforme, primitive neuroectodermal tumor, medulloblastoma, and astrocytoma; Lynch syndrome–associated tumors, including colorectal carcinoma; and other tumors, which have included neuroblastoma and rhabdomyosarcoma.[126]

In several reports, the café-au-lait observed in children with CMMR-D have been described as having a "ragged-edge, slightly diffuse appearance," with irregular borders.[128–131] Axillary freckling has been described in some patients.[128,132–135] Skin-fold freckling has been noted in some affected children, and isolated patients with plexiform neurofibroma, cutaneous neurofibroma, Lisch nodules, and pseudarthrosis of the tibia have been reported.[132,136–138] NF1 gene evaluation for patients with CMMR-D has been negative.[133,134,139,140] In addition, 3 siblings with CMMR-D and biallelic MSH2 germline mutations and a single patient with biallelic MSH6 mutations who manifested both hyperpigmented and hypopigmented cutaneous macules and patches have been reported.[130,141]

Somatic inactivation of the NF1 gene through mismatch repair defects has been proposed to explain the occurrence of café-au-lait, skin-fold freckling, and other features of NF-1 in affected patients. The NF1 gene has been shown to be a mutational target in mismatch repair–deficient cells.[142]

Ring Chromosome Syndromes

Multiple café-au-lait have been reported in patients with ring chromosome syndromes involving chromosomes 7, 11, 12, 15, and 17.[143–150] These children tend to present with a variety of other congenital anomalies including facial dysmorphism, microcephaly, and clinodactyly, as well as with short stature and neurocognitive deficits.

TREATMENT

Treatment of café-au-lait is not required for medical reasons, but is often requested by patients and caregivers for cosmetic concerns, in particular with large, segmental café-au-lait or when café-au-lait are present on the face. There is no uniformly successful treatment modality for removing café-au-lait. Several medical lasers have been used for the treatment of café-au-lait, all with variable clinical results. Complications of laser surgery include discoloration of the skin and scarring, and recurrence after treatment is common. The Q-switched ruby laser, erbium:YAG laser, 1064-nm frequency-doubled Q-switched Nd:YAG laser, copper vapor laser, and 510 nm pulsed-dye laser have all been used.[151–160]

SUMMARY

Café-au-lait are common pigmented skin lesions in children. Although most café-au-lait present as 1 or 2 hyperpigmented macules or patches in an otherwise healthy child, the presence of multiple café-au-lait, large segmental café-au-lait, associated facial dysmorphism, other cutaneous anomalies, or unusual findings on physical examination should suggest the possibility of an associated syndrome. While NF-1 is the most common syndrome seen in children with multiple café-au-lait, other syndromes associated with one or more café-au-lait include McCune-Albright syndrome, Legius syndrome, Noonan syndrome, and other neuro-cardio-facial-cutaneous syndromes.

REFERENCES

1. Ortonne JP, Brocard E, Floret D, et al. [Diagnostic value of café-au-lait spots (author's transl)]. Ann Dermatol Venereol 1980;107:313 [in French].
2. De Schepper S, Boucneau J, Vander Haeghen Y, et al. Café-au-lait spots in neurofibromatosis type 1 and in healthy control individuals: hyperpigmentation of a different kind? Arch Dermatol Res 2006;297:439.
3. Kaufmann D, Krone W, Hochsattel R, et al. A cell culture study on melanocytes from patients with neurofibromatosis-1. Arch Dermatol Res 1989;281:510.
4. Alper J, Holmes LB, Mihm MC Jr. Birthmarks with serious medical significance: nevocullular nevi, sebaceous nevi, and multiple café au lait spots. J Pediatr 1979;95:696.
5. Alper JC, Holmes LB. The incidence and significance of birthmarks in a cohort of 4,641 newborns. Pediatr Dermatol 1983;1:58.
6. Whitehouse D. Diagnostic value of the café-au-lait spot in children. Arch Dis Child 1966;41:316.
7. Burwell RG, James NJ, Johnston DI. Café-au-lait spots in schoolchildren. Arch Dis Child 1982;57:631.
8. McLean DI, Gallagher RP. "Sunburn" freckles, café-au-lait macules, and other pigmented lesions of schoolchildren: the Vancouver Mole Study. J Am Acad Dermatol 1995;32:565.
9. Rivers JK, MacLennan R, Kelly JW, et al. The eastern Australian childhood nevus study: prevalence of atypical nevi, congenital nevus-like nevi, and other pigmented lesions. J Am Acad Dermatol 1995;32:957.
10. Sigg C, Pelloni F, Schnyder UW. Frequency of congenital nevi, nevi spili and café-au-lait spots and their relation to nevus count and skin complexion in 939 children. Dermatologica 1990;180:118.
11. Riccardi VM. Von Recklinghausen neurofibromatosis. N Engl J Med 1981;305:1617.
12. Ducker P, Pfeiff B, Pullmann H. [Malignant melanoma in café-au-lait spot]. Z Hautkr 1990;65:751 [in German].
13. Perkinson NG. Melanoma arising in a café au lait spot of neurofibromatosis. Am J Surg 1957;93:1018.
14. Korf BR. Diagnostic outcome in children with multiple café au lait spots. Pediatrics 1992;90:924.
15. Fois A, Calistri L, Balestri P, et al. Relationship between café-au-lait spots as the only symptom and peripheral neurofibromatosis (NF1): a follow-up study. Eur J Pediatr 1993;152:500.
16. Nunley KS, Gao F, Albers AC, et al. Predictive value of café au lait macules at initial consultation in the diagnosis of neurofibromatosis type 1. Arch Dermatol 2009;145:883.
17. Crowe FW, Schull WJ. Diagnostic importance of café-au-lait spot in neurofibromatosis. AMA Arch Intern Med 1953;91:758.
18. Gutmann DH, Aylsworth A, Carey JC, et al. The diagnostic evaluation and multidisciplinary management of neurofibromatosis 1 and neurofibromatosis 2. JAMA 1997;278:51.

19. Stumpf DA, Alksne JF, Annegers JF, et al. Neurofibromatosis. Conference statement. National Institutes of Health Consensus Development Conference. Arch Neurol 1988;45:575.

20. Listernick R, Ferner RE, Liu GT, et al. Optic pathway gliomas in neurofibromatosis-1: controversies and recommendations. Ann Neurol 2007;61:189.

21. Listernick R, Louis DN, Packer RJ, et al. Optic pathway gliomas in children with neurofibromatosis 1: consensus statement from the NF1 optic pathway glioma task force. Ann Neurol 1997;41:143.

22. DeBella K, Szudek J, Friedman JM. Use of the national institutes of health criteria for diagnosis of neurofibromatosis 1 in children. Pediatrics 2000;105:608.

23. Boyd KP, Korf BR, Theos A. Neurofibromatosis type 1. J Am Acad Dermatol 2009;61:1.

24. Listernick R, Charrow J. Neurofibromatosis-1 in childhood. Adv Dermatol 2004;20:75.

25. Williams VC, Lucas J, Babcock MA, et al. Neurofibromatosis type 1 revisited. Pediatrics 2009;123:124.

26. Obringer AC, Meadows AT, Zackai EH. The diagnosis of neurofibromatosis-1 in the child under the age of 6 years. Am J Dis Child 1989;143:717.

27. Rosser T, Packer RJ. Neurofibromas in children with neurofibromatosis 1. J Child Neurol 2002;17:585.

28. Tonsgard JH, Kwak SM, Short MP, et al. CT imaging in adults with neurofibromatosis-1: frequent asymptomatic plexiform lesions. Neurology 1998;50:1755.

29. Evans DG, Baser ME, McGaughran J, et al. Malignant peripheral nerve sheath tumours in neurofibromatosis 1. J Med Genet 2002;39:311.

30. Gutmann DH, Gurney JG, Shannon KM. Juvenile xanthogranuloma, neurofibromatosis 1, and juvenile chronic myeloid leukemia. Arch Dermatol 1996;132:1390.

31. Zvulunov A, Barak Y, Metzker A. Juvenile xanthogranuloma, neurofibromatosis, and juvenile chronic myelogenous leukemia. World statistical analysis. Arch Dermatol 1995;131:904.

32. Ferner RE. Neurofibromatosis 1 and neurofibromatosis 2: a twenty first century perspective. Lancet Neurol 2007;6:340.

33. Rosser TL, Vezina G, Packer RJ. Cerebrovascular abnormalities in a population of children with neurofibromatosis type 1. Neurology 2005;64:553.

34. Bader JL, Miller RW. Neurofibromatosis and childhood leukemia. J Pediatr 1978;92:925.

35. Matsui I, Tanimura M, Kobayashi N, et al. Neurofibromatosis type 1 and childhood cancer. Cancer 1993;72:2746.

36. McKeen EA, Bodurtha J, Meadows AT, et al. Rhabdomyosarcoma complicating multiple neurofibromatosis. J Pediatr 1978;93:992.

37. Miettinen M, Fetsch JF, Sobin LH, et al. Gastrointestinal stromal tumors in patients with neurofibromatosis 1: a clinicopathologic and molecular genetic study of 45 cases. Am J Surg Pathol 2006;30:90.

38. Stiller CA, Chessells JM, Fitchett M. Neurofibromatosis and childhood leukaemia/lymphoma: a population-based UKCCSG study. Br J Cancer 1994;70:969.

39. Walther MM, Herring J, Enquist E, et al. von Recklinghausen's disease and pheochromocytomas. J Urol 1999;162:1582.

40. Rosser T, Packer RJ. Intracranial neoplasms in children with neurofibromatosis 1. J Child Neurol 2002;17:630.

84. Abeliovich D, Gelman-Kohan Z, Silverstein S, et al. Familial café au lait spots: a variant of neurofibromatosis type 1. J Med Genet 1995;32:985.

85. Brunner HG, Hulsebos T, Steijlen PM, et al. Exclusion of the neurofibromatosis 1 locus in a family with inherited café-au-lait spots. Am J Med Genet 1993;46:472.

86. Charrow J, Listernick R, Ward K. Autosomal dominant multiple café-au-lait spots and neurofibromatosis-1: evidence of non-linkage. Am J Med Genet 1993;45:606.

87. Riccardi VM. Pathophysiology of neurofibromatosis. IV. Dermatologic insights into heterogeneity and pathogenesis. J Am Acad Dermatol 1980;3:157.

88. Brems H, Chmara M, Sahbatou M, et al. Germline loss-of-function mutations in SPRED1 cause a neurofibromatosis 1-like phenotype. Nat Genet 2007;39:1120.

89. Wakioka T, Sasaki A, Kato R, et al. Spred is a Sprouty-related suppressor of Ras signalling. Nature 2001;412:647.

90. Pasmant E, Sabbagh A, Hanna N, et al. SPRED1 germline mutations caused a neurofibromatosis type 1 overlapping phenotype. J Med Genet 2009;46:425.

91. Messiaen L, Yao S, Brems H, et al. Clinical and mutational spectrum of neurofibromatosis type 1-like syndrome. JAMA 2009;302:2111.

92. Evans DG, Moran A, King A, et al. Incidence of vestibular schwannoma and neurofibromatosis 2 in the North West of England over a 10-year period: higher incidence than previously thought. Otol Neurotol 2005;26:93.

93. Evans DG, Huson SM, Donnai D, et al. A genetic study of type 2 neurofibromatosis in the United Kingdom. I. Prevalence, mutation rate, fitness, and confirmation of maternal transmission effect on severity. J Med Genet 1992;29:841.

94. Mautner VF, Lindenau M, Baser ME, et al. Skin abnormalities in neurofibromatosis 2. Arch Dermatol 1997;133:1539.

95. Parry DM, Eldridge R, Kaiser-Kupfer MI, et al. Neurofibromatosis 2 (NF2): clinical characteristics of 63 affected individuals and clinical evidence for heterogeneity. Am J Med Genet 1994;52:450.

96. Evans DG, Baser ME, O'Reilly B, et al. Management of the patient and family with neurofibromatosis 2: a consensus conference statement. Br J Neurosurg 2005;19:5.

97. Asthagiri AR, Parry DM, Butman JA, et al. Neurofibromatosis type 2. Lancet 2009;373:1974.

98. Ruggieri M, Iannetti P, Polizzi A, et al. Earliest clinical manifestations and natural history of neurofibromatosis type 2 (NF2) in childhood: a study of 24 patients. Neuropediatrics 2005;36:21.

99. Evans DG, Birch JM, Ramsden RT. Paediatric presentation of type 2 neurofibromatosis. Arch Dis Child 1999;81:496.

100. MacCollin M, Mautner VF. The diagnosis and management of neurofibromatosis 2 in childhood. Semin Pediatr Neurol 1998;5:243.

101. Nunes F, MacCollin M. Neurofibromatosis 2 in the pediatric population. J Child Neurol 2003;18:718.

102. Rouleau GA, Merel P, Lutchman M, et al. Alteration in a new gene encoding a putative membrane-organizing protein causes neuro-fibromatosis type 2. Nature 1993;363:515.

103. Trofatter JA, MacCollin MM, Rutter JL, et al. A novel moesin-, ezrin-, radixin-like gene is a candidate for the neurofibromatosis 2 tumor suppressor. Cell 1993;72:791.

104. Evans DG, Wallace AJ, Wu CL, et al. Somatic mosaicism: a common cause of classic disease in tumor-prone syndromes? Lessons from type 2 neurofibromatosis. Am J Hum Genet 1998;63:727.

105. Evans DG, Trueman L, Wallace A, et al. Genotype/phenotype correlations in type 2 neurofibromatosis (NF2): evidence for more severe disease associated with truncating mutations. J Med Genet 1998;35:450.

106. Albright F, Butler AM, Hampton AO, et al. Syndrome characterized by osteitis fibrosa disseminata, areas of pigmentation and endocrine dysfunction, with precocious puberty in females: report of five cases. N Engl J Med 1937;216:727.

107. Hogeling M, Frieden IJ. Segmental pigmentation disorder. Br J Dermatol 2010; 162:1337.

108. McCune DJ. Osteitis fibrosa cystica; the case of a nine year old girl who also exhibits precocious puberty, multiple pigmentation of the skin and hyperthyroidism. Am J Dis Child 1936;52:743.

109. Lumbroso S, Paris F, Sultan C. McCune-Albright syndrome: molecular genetics. J Pediatr Endocrinol Metab 2002;15(Suppl 3):875.

110. Ringel MD, Schwindinger WF, Levine MA. Clinical implications of genetic defects in G proteins. The molecular basis of McCune-Albright syndrome and Albright hereditary osteodystrophy. Medicine (Baltimore) 1996;75:171.

111. Albers N, Jorgens S, Deiss D, et al. McCune-Albright syndrome—the German experience. J Pediatr Endocrinol Metab 2002;15(Suppl 3):897.

112. de Sanctis C, Lala R, Matarazzo P, et al. McCune-Albright syndrome: a longitudinal clinical study of 32 patients. J Pediatr Endocrinol Metab 1999;12:817.

113. Lumbroso S, Paris F, Sultan C. Activating Gsalpha mutations: analysis of 113 patients with signs of McCune-Albright syndrome—a European Collaborative Study. J Clin Endocrinol Metab 2004;89:2107.

114. Diaz A, Danon M, Crawford J. McCune-Albright syndrome and disorders due to activating mutations of GNAS1. J Pediatr Endocrinol Metab 2007;20:853.

115. Lala R, Matarazzo P, Andreo M, et al. Impact of endocrine hyperfunction and phosphate wasting on bone in McCune-Albright syndrome. J Pediatr Endocrinol Metab 2002;15(Suppl 3):913.

116. Shenker A, Weinstein LS, Moran A, et al. Severe endocrine and nonendocrine manifestations of the McCune-Albright syndrome associated with activating mutations of stimulatory G protein GS. J Pediatr 1993;123:509.

117. Benedict PH, Szabo G, Fitzpatrick TB, et al. Melanotic macules in Albright's syndrome and in neurofibromatosis. JAMA 1968;205:618.

118. Happle R. The McCune-Albright syndrome: a lethal gene surviving by mosaicism. Clin Genet 1986;29:321.

119. Bowerman JE. Polyostotic fibrous dysplasia with oral melanotic pigmentation. Br J Oral Surg 1969;6:188.

120. Gorlin RJ, Chaudhry AP. Oral melanotic pigmentation in polyostotic fibrous dysplasia, Albright's syndrome. Oral Surg Oral Med Oral Pathol 1957;10:857.

121. Schwindinger WF, Francomano CA, Levine MA. Identification of a mutation in the gene encoding the alpha subunit of the stimulatory G protein of adenylyl cyclase in McCune-Albright syndrome. Proc Natl Acad Sci U S A 1992;89:5152.

122. Weinstein LS, Shenker A, Gejman PV, et al. Activating mutations of the stimulatory G protein in the McCune-Albright syndrome. N Engl J Med 1991;325:1688.

123. Donovan S, Shannon KM, Bollag G. GTPase activating proteins: critical regulators of intracellular signaling. Biochim Biophys Acta 2002;1602:23.

124. Weinstein LS. G(s)alpha mutations in fibrous dysplasia and McCune-Albright syndrome. J Bone Miner Res 2006;21(Suppl 2):P120.

125. Kim IS, Kim ER, Nam HJ, et al. Activating mutation of GS alpha in McCune-Albright syndrome causes skin pigmentation by tyrosinase gene activation on affected melanocytes. Horm Res 1999;52:235.

126. Wimmer K, Etzler J. Constitutional mismatch repair-deficiency syndrome: have we so far seen only the tip of an iceberg? Hum Genet 2008;124:105.
127. Lynch HT, de la Chapelle A. Hereditary colorectal cancer. N Engl J Med 2003; 348:919.
128. De Vos M, Hayward BE, Charlton R, et al. PMS2 mutations in childhood cancer. J Natl Cancer Inst 2006;98:358.
129. Kruger S, Kinzel M, Walldorf C, et al. Homozygous PMS2 germline mutations in two families with early-onset haematological malignancy, brain tumours, HNPCC-associated tumours, and signs of neurofibromatosis type 1. Eur J Hum Genet 2008;16:62.
130. Scott RH, Mansour S, Pritchard-Jones K, et al. Medulloblastoma, acute myelocytic leukemia and colonic carcinomas in a child with biallelic MSH6 mutations. Nat Clin Pract Oncol 2007;4:130.
131. Tan TY, Orme LM, Lynch E, et al. Biallelic PMS2 mutations and a distinctive childhood cancer syndrome. J Pediatr Hematol Oncol 2008;30:254.
132. Gallinger S, Aronson M, Shayan K, et al. Gastrointestinal cancers and neurofibromatosis type 1 features in children with a germline homozygous MLH1 mutation. Gastroenterology 2004;126:576.
133. Hegde MR, Chong B, Blazo ME, et al. A homozygous mutation in MSH6 causes Turcot syndrome. Clin Cancer Res 2005;11:4689.
134. Ostergaard JR, Sunde L, Okkels H. Neurofibromatosis von Recklinghausen type I phenotype and early onset of cancers in siblings compound heterozygous for mutations in MSH6. Am J Med Genet A 2005;139A:96.
135. Vilkki S, Tsao JL, Loukola A, et al. Extensive somatic microsatellite mutations in normal human tissue. Cancer Res 2001;61:4541.
136. Raevaara TE, Gerdes AM, Lonnqvist KE, et al. HNPCC mutation MLH1 P648S makes the functional protein unstable, and homozygosity predisposes to mild neurofibromatosis type 1. Genes Chromosomes Cancer 2004;40:261.
137. Ricciardone MD, Ozcelik T, Cevher B, et al. Human MLH1 deficiency predisposes to hematological malignancy and neurofibromatosis type 1. Cancer Res 1999;59:290.
138. Wang Q, Lasset C, Desseigne F, et al. Neurofibromatosis and early onset of cancers in hMLH1-deficient children. Cancer Res 1999;59:294.
139. Menko FH, Kaspers GL, Meijer GA, et al. A homozygous MSH6 mutation in a child with café-au-lait spots, oligodendroglioma and rectal cancer. Fam Cancer 2004;3:123.
140. Trimbath JD, Petersen GM, Erdman SH, et al. Café-au-lait spots and early onset colorectal neoplasia: a variant of HNPCC? Fam Cancer 2001;1:101.
141. Scott RH, Homfray T, Huxter NL, et al. Familial T-cell non-Hodgkin lymphoma caused by biallelic MSH2 mutations. J Med Genet 2007;44:e83.
142. Wang Q, Montmain G, Ruano E, et al. Neurofibromatosis type 1 gene as a mutational target in a mismatch repair-deficient cell type. Hum Genet 2003;112:117.
143. Fagan K, Suthers GK, Hardacre G. Ring chromosome 11 and café-au-lait spots. Am J Med Genet 1988;30:911.
144. Morava E, Bartsch O, Czako M, et al. A girl with cutaneous hyperpigmentation, café au lait spots and ring chromosome 15 without significant deletion. Genet Couns 2003;14:337.
145. Park JP, Graham JM Jr, Andrews PA, et al. Ring chromosome 12. Am J Med Genet 1988;29:437.
146. Shashi V, White JR, Pettenati MJ, et al. Ring chromosome 17: phenotype variation by deletion size. Clin Genet 2003;64:361.

147. Surace C, Piazzolla S, Sirleto P, et al. Mild ring 17 syndrome shares common phenotypic features irrespective of the chromosomal breakpoints location. Clin Genet 2009;76:256.
148. Vollenweider Roten S, Masouye I, Delozier-Blanchet CD, et al. Cutaneous findings in ring chromosome 7 syndrome. Dermatology 1993;186:84.
149. Wahlstrom J, Bjarnason R, Rosdahl I, et al. Boy with a ring 7 chromosome: a case report with special reference to dermatological findings. Acta Paediatr 1996;85:1256.
150. Zen PR, Pinto LL, Graziadio C, et al. Association of microcephaly and café-au-lait spots in a patient with ring chromosome 12 syndrome. Clin Dysmorphol 2005;14:141.
151. Alora MB, Arndt KA. Treatment of a café-au-lait macule with the erbium:YAG laser. J Am Acad Dermatol 2001;45:566.
152. Alster TS. Complete elimination of large café-au-lait birthmarks by the 510-nm pulsed dye laser. Plast Reconstr Surg 1995;96:1660.
153. Alster TS, Williams CM. Café-au-lait macule in type V skin: successful treatment with a 510 nm pulsed dye laser. J Am Acad Dermatol 1995;33:1042.
154. Carpo BG, Grevelink JM, Grevelink SV. Laser treatment of pigmented lesions in children. Semin Cutan Med Surg 1999;18:233.
155. Idorn LW, Haedersdal M. Paradoxical postoperative hyperpigmentation from Q-switched YAG laser treatment of pigmented lesions in children with fair skin types. J Eur Acad Dermatol Venereol 2009;23:856.
156. Kim JS, Kim MJ, Cho SB. Treatment of segmental café-au-lait macules using 1064-nm Q-switched Nd:YAG laser with low pulse energy. Clin Exp Dermatol 2009;34:e223.
157. Nelson JS, Applebaum J. Treatment of superficial cutaneous pigmented lesions by melanin-specific selective photothermolysis using the Q-switched ruby laser. Ann Plast Surg 1992;29:231.
158. Shimbashi T, Kamide R, Hashimoto T. Long-term follow-up in treatment of solar lentigo and café-au-lait macules with Q-switched ruby laser. Aesthetic Plast Surg 1997;21:445.
159. Somyos K, Boonchu K, Somsak K, et al. Copper vapour laser treatment of café-au-lait macules. Br J Dermatol 1996;135:964.
160. Tse Y, Levine VJ, McClain SA, et al. The removal of cutaneous pigmented lesions with the Q-switched ruby laser and the Q-switched neodymium: yttrium-aluminum-garnet laser. A comparative study. J Dermatol Surg Oncol 1994;20:795.

Congenital Melanocytic Nevi

Valerie B. Lyon, MD

KEYWORDS

- Nevus • Congenital nevus • Congenital melanocytic nevus
- Pigmented nevus • Garmet nevus • Giant nevus
- Melanocytic nevus • Childhood melanoma

One of the most common skin lesions in a newborn infant is the congenital melanocytic nevus. These lesions pose considerable clinical dilemma given their frequency, wide variation in presentation, potential psychosocial impact, and potential for medical significance. All of these factors affect decisions regarding their treatment. In general, lesions are either observed or removed with excisional surgery. Occasionally intermediary procedures, such as biopsy or alternative surgical procedure, are considered. A congenital nevus on a child can be a source of anxiety and distress for parents. The medical significance of these newborn skin lesions is that over a lifetime they can be a marker for increased risk of malignancy, may be associated with rare syndromes, or can transform into melanoma. Thankfully, melanoma in children is rare. Nonetheless, it does occur and the risk for melanoma increases dramatically at puberty.

The relative risk for melanoma arising within a congenital nevus is related to the size of the lesion. The timing of and clinical presentation of development of melanoma is also related to the size of the lesion. Medical decisions are individualized taking into account the perceived risk of malignancy, psychosocial impact, and anticipated treatment outcome. In this chapter, the common features of congenital nevi are discussed as well as the potential individual variations and their impact on treatment recommendations.

DEFINITION AND CLASSIFICATION

A congenital melanocytic nevus is composed of melanocytes, the pigment-forming cells in the skin. This is in contrast to the broader category of congenital "nevi," which may include nevus sebaceous (sebaceous gland proliferation) and epidermal nevus (keratinocyte proliferation). In contrast to acquired melanocytic nevi, congenital melanocytic nevi are present on the skin at birth or within the first year of life. A tardive

---

Department of Dermatology, Medical College of Wisconsin, 9200 West Wisconsin Avenue, Milwaukee, WI 53226, USA
E-mail address: vlyon@mcw.edu

Pediatr Clin N Am 57 (2010) 1155–1176
doi:10.1016/j.pcl.2010.07.005
0031-3955/10/$ – see front matter © 2010 Elsevier Inc. All rights reserved.

pediatric.theclinics.com

congenital nevus is one that is not present at birth but becomes clinically apparent within the first 2 to 3 years of life. Congenital melanocytic nevi are considered benign nevomelanocytic proliferations and are common, with estimates in prevalence at 1% to 6%.[1–5]

At birth, the lesions may be lightly pigmented macules or patches that in some cases mimic café au lait macules. They may be pink at birth, as is more typical on the scalp, or multiple shades of brown black. They are commonly small and oval, but can be a range of sizes and unlimited potential shapes, with round, linear, curvilinear, geographic pattern and random shape among the most common forms. Multiple lesions can be found, coalescing on one anatomic area, discontinuous in a geographic area, or randomly scattered. Once fully developed, the typical appearance is that of a pigmented brown plaque that is round to oval in shape, with regular, smooth, and well-demarcated borders. In addition to variations in shape, the fully formed congenital melanocytic nevus can have variations in border and coloration such as ill-defined, fading borders that are shades of brown, areas of darker brown or black pigmentation either symmetrically in the center of the lesion or randomly distributed within the lesion. Variations can also occur in surface characteristics and nevi can have a pebbly or rough surface or extremely hyperkeratotic surface, and frequently exhibit hypertrichosis. Most congenial melanocytic nevi occur sporadically but familial clustering has been observed.[6]

Treatment depends on the location, size, appearance, and symptoms of the lesion; parental concerns; and presence of other risk factors.

The most commonly used classification for congenital melanocytic nevi is based on size with small (<1.5 cm), medium (1.5–19 cm), and large (>20 cm) lesions defined by the largest dimension diameter anticipated in *adulthood*.[7]

The term giant congenital nevus is used for nevi covering large segments of the body. Other classifications that have less commonly been used for congenital nevi include those based on relationship to an anatomic structure (palm-size multiples),[8] ease of removal (requiring skin graft),[9,10] and relative body surface area (BSA) of involvement (30% BSA significance).[11]

In infants and children, classification according to size is based on eventual anticipated size, and thus lesions on the head greater than 9 cm or on the body greater than 6 cm in an infant are referred to as large congenital nevi because relative eventual growth to approximately1.5 times and 3.0 times the size occurs on the head or body, respectively.[12–14]

Recently, a proposed refinement in classification recommends separating medium from large congenital melanocytic nevi (CMN) at 10 and 20 cm, respectively, and defining a giant CMN as one measuring more than 20 cm in greatest diameter.[15]

In this classification, giant lesions are further recognized in 10-cm intervals (G1, G2, G3), and in patients with more than 50 satellite lesions, the size category is increased by one category to account for the increased risk of melanoma. This classification allows for more precise stratification according to size and therefore nevus burden. Since as a general principle with CMN, size correlates with the depth of the lesion into the subcutis and with the total number of melanocytes present in the lesion.

Clinical appearance has not been considered a classifying feature for congenital nevi but is important for assessment of malignant potential, with and without regard to size. Uniformity and symmetry of coloration, shape, border, and topography are important clinical distinctions and will be reviewed later. A homogeneous uniform color and symmetric shape CMN with uniform topography (eg, no distinct papules) (**Fig. 1**) is less concerning than a multicolored CMN with an uneven surface and (**Fig. 2**) with irregular borders.

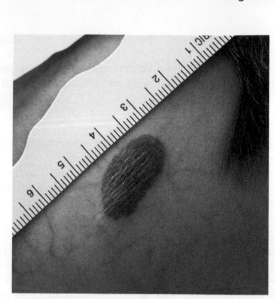

Fig. 1. Typical CMN.

Synonyms for CMN include garment nevus, bathing trunk nevus, giant hairy nevus, giant pigmented nevus, pigmented hairy nevus, nevus pigmentosus, nevus pigmentosus et pilosus, and Tierfell nevus. Nevus spilus, which is characterized by a café-au-lait–like macule or patch with speckled pigmented macules and papules within it, may represent a clinical variant of congenital melanocytic nevus, especially when papular areas are present within the lesion (nevus spilus papulosis).[16,17]

Tardive congenital nevi are nevi with congenital features that are not present at birth but instead arise within the first 1 to 2 years of life.

The term congenital-nevus–like nevus refers to a pigmented nevus that was not reported to be present at birth or shortly thereafter; however, it has histologic features consistent with a congenital nevus. It is unknown whether these represent congenital nevi that were present but not externally visible until later or whether these are actually acquired nevi with congenital histologic features. The prevalence of congenital-nevus–like nevus is estimated at 2% to 6% of the population. The term early-onset nevus has also been used.

PATHOGENESIS

The cause of congenital nevi is not known. In normal human development in utero, melanocytes are derived from the neural crest as melanoblasts and migrate from a dorsal location in the embryo ventrally to the skin, the central nervous system (CNS), eye, and adrenal glands between weeks 5 and 24 of gestation. Defects in migration or maturation are hypothesized. The molecular[18,19] and genetic changes

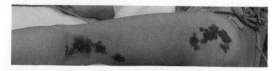

Fig. 2. CMN with pigment, border, texture, and shape irregularity.

and chromosomal aberrations in congenital nevi are beginning to be characterized.[20–22]

Somatic mosaicism and clonality have been suggested given the repetitive patterns of occurrence along developmental skin lines and the observation of twin spots.[23]

CLINICAL PRESENTATION

Congenital nevi may have many different appearances in coloration, topography, and border, but the shape and pattern are often repetitive.[24]

The congenital nevus is usually a round to oval shape and may be oriented with the long axis along lines of skin development (**Fig. 3**). The color is usually brown to dark brown or black plaque with a rugose or mamillated topography.

Coloration

In the first few years of life, the lesions can be flat and less heavily pigmented color, and the appearance can mimic that of a café au lait macule (**Fig. 4**). Occasionally congenital nevi, especially those located on the scalp and face can be pink-red and rarely without color (nonpigmented) (**Fig. 5**).[25,26] Rarely lesions may become hypopigmented or even regress.[27–31]

More than one color can be present in a congenital nevus and most frequently are shades of brown and dark brown or black. The coloration can be present in a speckled pattern with darker brown papules randomly scattered in a tan-colored macular background (nevus spilus papulosis or speckled congenital nevus),[32,33] or irregularly, randomly distributed papules or nodules in larger lesions.[34]

The border of the nevus can be a different hue from the central body of the nevus, resembling a fried egg if darker color centrally than at the periphery, or, if lighter centrally and darker on the border, can resemble an eclipse. When congenital nevi consist of a predominantly pink color, they can have overlying hyperkeratosis and mimic a plaque of eczema.

On occasion, congenital nevi are not present at birth because the melanocytes lack visible pigment. In these cases, the CMN becomes clinically apparent within the first 2 years of life and is referred to as a "tardive" congenital nevus. In the case of a melanocytic nevus mimicking the appearance of a café au lait macule with tan brown color

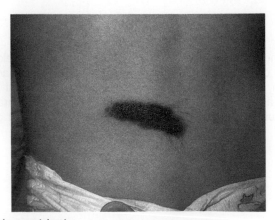

Fig. 3. CMN with hypertrichosis.

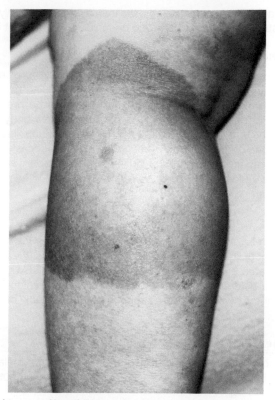

Fig. 4. CMN mimicking a café au lait macule. (*Courtesy of* Liborka Kos, MD.)

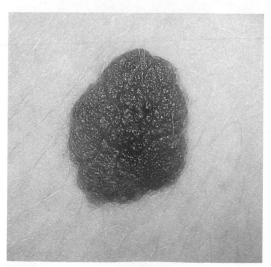

Fig. 5. CMN with pink color.

and macular instead of plaque morphology, the lesion thickens usually over a period of years, and the distinction toward true nevus becomes more evident in this time.

Shape and Configuration

Nevoid shape is generally oval, but round, geographic, curvilinear, arcuate, ink blot, leaflike, and more angular shapes such as square, rectangular, or triangular shapes can be seen. When multiple lesions are present, they can be present in the same anatomic segment or area or be randomly distributed on the body. When localized to one segment of the body, multiple lesions can be discontinuous in a random pattern or coalescing into one of the previously mentioned shapes, occasionally background tan coloration encompasses the group of individual nevi. Borders can be well defined or ill defined, can be uniform and regular, or can be irregular—either uniformly irregular or randomly irregular.

Location

Congenital nevi can involve any location in the skin including the mouth, palms and soles, and nails (**Fig. 6**).[35] When located in the mouth and nails, the lesions are usually macular. When located on the scalp, the lesion commonly displays a central area of coloration that is a different shade or color than the rim. Benign features of these lesions are symmetry of shape and pigmentation and a lack of other significant irregularities.

Secondary Changes

Although the surface is typically rugose and elevated, congenital melanocytic nevi can be flat, especially in the first 1 to 2 years of life. Randomly distributed papules may

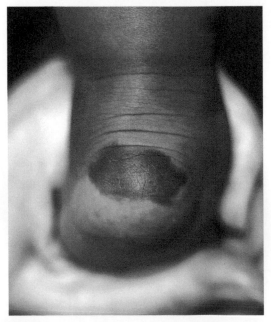

Fig. 6. Acral congenital nevus.

occur within an otherwise flat lesion. Alternatively, the entire lesion can be significantly elevated off the skin surface, resembling a tumorlike growth. Congenital melanocytic nevi frequently develop hypertrichosis (symmetric) over the surface and frequently this hair is hyperpigmented as well. This can be especially dramatic in the scalp where congenital nevi can have hypertrichosis as well as hyperpigmentation of the scalp hair in the area. As previously mentioned, eczemalike appearance resulting from hyperkeratosis is common. Very thick hyperkeratosis resembling an epidermal nevus can also occur. Erosion and ulceration of the surface can be found. Heavily pigmented large congenital melanocytic nevi over a limb may be found in association with under-development of the limb, resulting in limb asymmetry.

Within an individual CMN, multiple variations in any of the previously mentioned descriptive characteristics can coexist.

Multiplicity

One lesion is normally present, but multiple congenital nevi can be present in the same patient, numbering hundreds. "Satellite nevi" describes the presence of multiple small congenital nevi in association with a large congenital nevus (**Fig. 7**).

CLINICAL COURSE

Congenital nevi will often "fill in" in the first few years of life. A once ill-defined border may become more defined and color may darken. They tend to thicken over a period of years. On the contrary, however, lesions may lighten over time as well and some lesions may even regress, especially in patients with vitiligo. The lesions can develop hypertrichosis, which, when uniformly distributed, is considered a normal occurrence. Hyperkeratosis can develop over the lesion secondary to dryness or concomitant eczema. Lesions once homogeneous can become speckled and lesions once flat can become papular or proliferative nodules can develop (**Figs. 8** and **9**). In the first few years of life some lesions can grow rapidly,[14] but many are assumed to grow pro-portionately with the growth of the child. Erosions[36] or proliferative nodules can occur within the first few weeks of life and although they should be considered a potential sign of malignancy, this can be a normal occurrence as well.

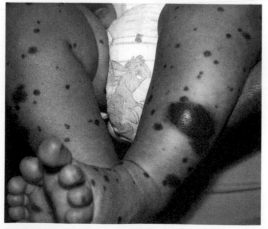

Fig. 7. Multiple satellite congenital nevi. (*Courtesy of* Liborka Kos, MD.)

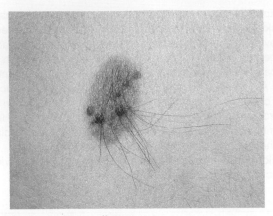

Fig. 8. Papules developing within small CMN.

DIAGNOSIS

Diagnosis of a congenital nevus is usually a clinical diagnosis made by history of the nevus since birth and the distinctive clinical appearance of that of a larger nevus that has a rugose topography (see **Fig. 2**). Diagnosis can be verified via skin biopsy, when necessary, which usually demonstrates typical histologic features.

HISTOLOGY

CMNs display characteristic histology including infiltration into the reticular dermis (and occasionally in the subcutaneous tissue including muscle and nerves extending in the subfascial plane), infiltration in and around skin appendages including hair follicles and sweat glands, and infiltration of single cells or single file between collagen bundles.[37]

In giant congenital nevi, nevus cells have been found infiltrating the blood vessels and lymphatics. Although the vast majority of congenital nevi share these features, some truly congenital nevi that are small may not display this histology. Many different

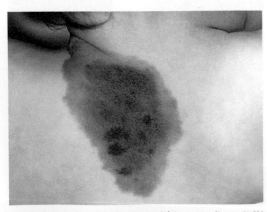

Fig. 9. Multiple pigmented macules developing within a medium CMN.

histologic subtypes of congenital nevi exist[30,38–42] with junctional, deep, blue, combined, and Spitz representing some of the more common descriptive subsets.

The misdiagnosis of pigmented lesions is common and they can often be difficult to distinguish from other entities. For this reason, histologic interpretation of congenital melanocytic nevi that are atypical or questionable should be made by a pathologist experienced in the interpretation of pigmented skin lesions.[38,43,44]

SIGNIFICANCE

A congenital nevus can have medical, cosmetic, and psychological implications. Congenital melanocytic nevi have been associated with the presence of other congenital skin lesions as well as random internal associations.[33,45–49]

Presence of congenital nevi as part of the NAME (LAMB or Carney) syndrome has been described.[50]

Malignancy has been reported in increased frequency within these lesions including melanoma and rhabdomyosarcoma,[51] liposarcoma, and peripheral nerve sheath tumor. The most significant feature of a congenital nevus is the associated risk for transformation into malignant melanoma.[38,52–61]

Although the exact risk of transformation is unknown, estimates for risk of transformation vary and the lifetime risk ranges from 4% to 10%. Smaller lesions are thought to have lower risk for transformation than larger congenital nevi[62] relative to the "nevus burden." The risk for small CMN is controversial and is thought to be between and 0% and 4.0%,[9,14,63,64] and for those with large or giant CMN the risk estimates are between 4.5% and 10.0%.[62,65–71]

Earlier estimates that were higher (as high as 42%) are now thought to be flawed from methodology or lack of improved histology. Although there are multiple reports of melanoma arising in small congenital nevi, studies fail to show an overall increased risk in this subset. Many of these small lesions are removed earlier in life before the onset for the greatest risk of melanoma; the impact of this on the natural history is unknown.

Melanoma arising from large congenital nevi presents in a different manner in large congenital nevi than in small congenital nevi.[72,73] Melanoma typically presents at a very young age (first 2–5 years of life) in these larger lesions. Seventy percent of patients with a large CMN diagnosed with melanoma are diagnosed within the first 10 years of life.[69]

Melanoma most commonly begins in deeper dermis or subcutaneous tissue in larger lesions and therefore often presents as a palpable nodule. Patients with melanoma in early childhood may be diagnosed with melanoma of unknown primary origin site because the focus of melanoma is hidden somewhere deep in the skin or subcutaneous tissue and cannot be found. Melanoma that is deep to the surface of the skin may be difficult to find in these larger lesions. Melanoma associated with these lesions may alternatively present outside of the involved skin and instead within the associated areas of neurocutaneous melanocytosis in the central nervous system.

Smaller lesions of congenital nevi are thinner in their depth of penetration into the skin and thus melanocytic aberrations occur in the superficial skin layers (at the dermal epidermal junction rather than in the subcutis). The transformation into melanoma is more commonly noticed as a change in pigmentation and/or shape of the lesion. The most frequent presentation is an area of hypopigmentation (or hyperpigmentation) on the periphery of the lesion.[74,75] In these smaller congenital melanocytic nevi, the development of melanoma more often is not until adulthood, perhaps related to the smaller burden of nevus cells and therefore less cell cycle activity.

In addition to being precursors to melanoma, the presence of a CMN may be a risk factor for the eventual development of melanoma anywhere on the skin, not necessarily within the lesion. The presence of a congenital nevus has been associated with an increase in the development of melanoma over a lifetime.[76] Some investigators think this is controversial.[76]

Parental anxiety can also be significant in patients with congenital nevi. Anxiety is expected regarding potential development of skin cancer in pigmented lesions; however, beyond the risk of cancer, the presence of a congenital nevus can contribute to anxiety because of the social stigmatization from the visual presence of a lesion that is different or disfiguring, anxiety regarding changes within a lesion, requirements for increased sun precautions, knowledge of risk of associated conditions such as neurocutaneous melanocytosis, or pain or discomfort associated with multiple medical procedures or scars. Behavioral changes have been found in as many as 30% of children with a large CMN, which may result from or contribute to family stress.[77]

NEUROCUTANEOUS MELANOCYTOSIS

Neurocutaneous melanocytosis is a rare syndrome of increased melanocytes in the CNS in the presence of congenital nevus on the skin. The first historical classification in 1972 defined the condition as having (1) large or numerous pigmented nevi in association with leptomeningeal melanocytosis or melanoma, (2) no evidence of malignancy in any of the skin lesions, and (3) no evidence of melanoma in any location other than the meninges.[78] The criteria have been refined more recently to the widely accepted definition of (1) the presence of a large CMN (>9 cm on the head or 6 cm on the body) or multiple (more than 3) congenital melanocytic nevi on the skin; (2) no evidence of cutaneous melanoma, except in people without meningeal melanoma as proven by biopsy; and (3) no evidence of meningeal melanoma, except in patients with benign cutaneous histology (also proven by histology).[79] Whereas the presence of increased melanocytes in the CNS may indicate proliferation of benign melanocytes (neurocutaneous melanocytosis [NCM]) or malignant melanocytes (primary melanoma or metastatic melanoma [MM]), neurocutaneous melanocytosis refers to the presence of an increased number of melanocytes in the CNS or meninges without melanoma. Melanocytes are present normally in the CNS, but in the presence of NCM, they are increased in number and usually associated with the existence of a CMN. Although the exact incidence of NCM is unknown, this is a rare phenomenon.

NCM can be asymptomatic or symptomatic. Symptomatic NCM is associated with a grave prognosis, and thus it is important to screen all at-risk patients for symptoms of NCM. Proliferation of melanocytes in the CNS can result in a variety of complications depending on the location of the melanocytes, including obstruction of cerebrospinal fluid, compression of vital structures, and even death.

The risk for associated NCM in a patient with a congenital nevus is thought to be greater in patients with large lesions,[79,80] which, as previously defined, includes those that are anticipated to be greater than 9 cm on the head or 6 cm on the body. In patients with large CMN, the subgroup of patients with a large CMN in an anatomic location that is posterior (eg, the posterior head, neck, spine, or paravertebral location) are the patients most likely to have associated NCM, and especially those with multiple satellite nevi.[79,80]

It is important to recognize that even patients with multiple medium-sized congenital nevi are also at risk for NCM, as are those with multiple satellite (small) CMN (>3) without a large nevus.[79]

Diagnosis of neurocutaneous melanocytosis is made by magnetic resonance imaging.[81,82]

Increased melanin is detected most commonly in the cerebellum or anterior temporal lobes and manifests with thickening of the leptomeninges and/or T1 (less likely T2) shortening in the brain parenchyma or meninges. Findings can be subtle and difficult to interpret and experience in interpreting the radiologic findings in these lesions is necessary.

NCM usually presents in the first few years of life, with rare cases reported in the second or fourth decade. Although most patients with NCM are asymptomatic, symptoms may include seizures, hydrocephalus, developmental delay, motor delay, nerve damage or spinal cord compression, or impaired mental status.[83] Symptomatic patients generally present earlier, within the first 2 years of life.

There is no standard recommended screening for NCM or follow-up interval. Patients planning complicated surgical resection of the CMN frequently undergo screening MRI. MRI before 4 months of age is more sensitive, because myelination of the CNS after that time can obscure subtle infiltrates. Approximately half of all patients with large CMN lesions were screened in a registry-based study.[84]

The interval for re-screening of positive patients is determined by the individual circumstances, such as extent of involvement of the melanocytosis and presence of neurologic symptoms. The necessity for follow-up MRI evaluation a patient with an initial negative screen is unknown. Although early MRI follow-up has been recommended for those with diagnosis of NCM, close neurologic follow-up seems to be a reasonable alternative, as current treatments are not curative and are directed toward relieving symptoms.

Treatments for neurocutaneous melanocytosis include those to control seizures, and/or interventions to relieve intracranial pressure, such as shunt placement, and those to stop proliferation of melanocytes. Combined chemotherapy and radiation has also been attempted but not met with much success. Unfortunately, interferon alpha and interleukin (IL)-2 have also been ineffective in treating melanoma in the CNS. Other chemotherapy agents are under investigation for CNS disease. Surgical resection has also been performed, although even with treatment, the prognosis is not altered.

Regarding the projected outcome for NCM, there are 2 prognostic categories: those with asymptomatic NCM and those with symptomatic NCM. For the vast majority of patients who have symptomatic NCM, the outcome has been fatal within a few years after diagnosis. Treatment in these cases is palliative. For patients with asymptomatic NCM, there is a wider spectrum and the prognosis is unknown.

Melanoma associated with a large congenital nevus may also occur in areas of neurocutaneous melanocytosis.

TREATMENT FOR CONGENITAL NEVI
Lesion Assessment

The treatment for a CMN is tailored to the individual patient.[85–87] Factors important in determining the treatment include symptoms associated with the lesion, size and appearance of the lesion, anatomic location of the lesion and ease of monitoring, psychosocial burden associated with the lesion, presence of risk factors for melanoma, and parental anxiety associated with the lesion.[88]

Indications for treatment exist on a continuum from very benign appearing lesions needing observation alone to significantly atypical appearing lesions according to the ABC guidelines (asymmetry, border irregularity, color asymmetry). Significant symptoms also include those used as guidelines for all melanocytic lesions, such as prolonged bleeding (longer than a 2-week period), itching, or growth out of proportion to the growth of the child. Significant deviation from the normal or change within a lesion can be an indication of the need for biopsy and/or removal. Excisional biopsy is the preferred procedure for accurate histopathologic diagnosis and prevention of future transformation. It should be kept in mind that even CMNs that are benign in appearance can have asymmetry of the shape, can have border irregularity, and can have even minimal color irregularity and therefore each lesion has to be considered with a knowledge of other risk factors and considerations for surgical treatment.

For congenital nevi, the larger the size of the lesion the greater the risk for melanoma is thought to be. In general, overall risk factors for melanoma include family history of melanoma or multiple atypical nevi, presence of risk factors in the patient's past medical history such as genetic predisposition to melanoma or previous cancer, and risk factors found on physical examination of the patient's skin with regard to sun phototype and other nevi (**Table 1**).

Anatomic location of the lesion with respect to whether it impedes long-term observation by the patient or is readily visible to the patient for examination is a factor in deciding treatment. Prophylactic removal is recommended in lesions located in an anatomic location that precludes observation such as the back, buttock, or scalp. Lesions that are thick, rugose, or heterogeneous can be difficult to monitor and removal should be considered. Lesions that are irregular with regard to coloration, texture, and/or shape may preclude meaningful observation for significant changes and should be considered for removal as well (see **Fig. 2**). Photographs of irregularly shaped or pigmented lesions can be very helpful in monitoring. The parent can be encouraged to take his or her own photograph for later comparison as well.

Clearly, lesions that are clinically very atypical warrant excisional biopsy. On the other hand, prophylactic removal of all normal-appearing CMNs, however, is not warranted. Surgical removal of small congenital nevi that become symptomatic justify excisional biopsy. A congenital nevus that is located in an anatomic position that prevents observation over a lifetime may justify the removal of an otherwise benign-appearing small congenital nevus, especially in the presence of other risk factors for melanoma. Lager lesions have greater risk for the development for melanoma and are, therefore, frequently removed even when less clinically atypical. Although surgical removal can effectively reduce the lesions, it should be remembered that it is nearly

Table 1				
Risk factors for melanoma				
	Melanoma	**Nevi**	**Physical Examination**	**Other Medical History**
Patient	Personal history of melanoma	Presence of multiple nevi Presence of atypical or large nevi (Clark's or dysplastic nevi)	Red hair Blue eyes Freckling Multiple nevi Atypical nevi (sun-sensitive phototype)	History of nonmelanoma skin cancer, history of cancer, non-skin related, history of radiation or chemotherapy, immunosuppression, immunodeficiency
Family	First- or second-degree relative with melanoma	Family history of multiple atypical nevi and patient presence of atypical nevus		

impossible, however, to completely remove all the nevus cells associated with giant CMNs. Patients and practitioners should be aware that the risk of melanoma can therefore never be completely mitigated. Additionally, some of these patients may develop melanoma in the CNS at an unrelated site.

Treatment Considerations

Surgical removal needs to be weighed in consideration for the likelihood of risk for impaired function resulting from surgery, likelihood for an improved cosmetic result, potential for uncomfortable scar, or complications from surgery including infection or bleeding.[77]

Surgical removal should also be weighed in consideration of resultant potential deformity of the anatomic area based on development or anatomy. A multispecialty approach with surgical input or consultation should be used for lesions that are in developmentally, cosmetically, or functionally significant locations and when lesions are large. A multidisciplinary approach with plastic surgery, dermatology, pathology, radiology and psychology can be helpful in extensive or difficult cases. For large nevi, serial surgeries may be required for removal of the lesion. Before surgical procedure, postsurgical expectations need to be realistic and should include discussion of the anticipated scar, surgical risks, recurrence along the scar line, and lack of complete removal of risk for melanoma development throughout life.

It should be kept in mind that surgical removal of a large CMN may lessen the tumor burden and is thereby assumed to decrease the risk for development of melanoma within the lesions. However, the absolute risk of melanoma in these lesions is unknown and controversial and well-designed randomized controlled trials for large or small congenital nevi have not been performed. Large, randomized controlled trials may never be performed for these lesions because small lesions are now more frequently removed because of ease of the procedure and larger lesions are frequently removed either partially or totally because of the symptoms or psychosocial burden associated with their presence. In addition, the use of tissue expanders and general anesthesia in children has expanded, allowing greater security in surgical treatment.

Observation

Observation without removal is warranted for benign-appearing small congenital nevi (see **Fig. 1**) or in cases where self-examination over a lifetime is feasible, where surgery is likely to result in functional impairment or disfiguring scarring or when potential complications of surgery outweigh the anticipated benefit, or parents (or patients of age) are morally opposed. There is no standard recommended interval for observation. The greater the atypia of the clinical appearance, the shorter the recommended interval between physician visits. A benign congenital melanocytic nevus that is small can be monitored by a physician on a yearly basis when available, and by patients, parents, or guardians on a more frequent basis; frequently, a monthly interval for home observation is recommended. With larger lesions, more frequent visits in the first 4 years of life are appropriate because most melanomas present in early childhood. Palpation of these larger lesions is important to assess for nodularity, which can represent a focus of melanoma. The assessment for neurologic signs of NCM is also important in patients with large lesions or other at-risk lesions as previously mentioned. In contrast, follow-up for smaller lesions is especially important after puberty when the risk for transformation is greater in these lesions, and this is when a heightened suspicion of symptoms or clinical changes is appropriate.

Parents and patients should be taught ABCD(E) (asymmetry, border irregularity, color irregularity, diameter >5mm, evolution) guidelines of signs and symptoms of melanoma. A photograph of the lesion can be very helpful to assess for slight changes within a lesion and because most homes now have cameras in some form, this should be recommended. Childhood melanoma is more often symptomatic with rapid increase in size, pruritus, change in color, palpable mass, pain, bleeding, and lymph node enlargement as potential signs at presentation.[73]

Thus, particular attention should be paid to these symptoms. Dermoscopy and confocal microscopy (where available) are additional diagnostic tools that can detect small foci of superficially located melanoma. Dermoscopy is an office technique of using a handheld reflectance microscope and is now used as an additional tool by many dermatology practitioners. Dermoscopy can be used to both identify and diagnose a congenital nevus and for closer inspection to evaluate for significant changes. Several different dermatoscopic patterns for CMNs have been described and the body of knowledge around its utility for CMN is growing.[1,89,90]

Clinical Course and Management

Frequently, congenital nevi develop new colors or new papules within them. Such changes can be benign or can signify malignant change. Treatment recommendations can include continued observation if the coloration or change is symmetric and changes cease. Removal can be complete via excision with biopsy, or if necessary for large lesions, biopsy can be performed from a representative area without complete removal. In general, excisional biopsy is the preferred method for sampling of a melanocytic lesion with changes suspicious for melanoma, as the histologic diagnosis of melanoma is based on the symmetry of the infiltrate of nevus cells over the breadth of the specimen as well as the microscopic architecture and the individual cellular characteristics.

The pathologic interpretation of the biopsy of a congenital melanocytic nevus should be interpreted by a clinician trained in evaluation of pigmented skin lesions. It should be remembered, however, than just as with common acquired melanocytic nevi, there is often a discordance between the clinical impression and the microscopic interpretation. Lesions that mimic melanoma clinically may be interpreted as benign with histopathology.[91]

Light microscopy is still the standard for interpretation of diagnosis. Special stains can be used in lesions to determine melanocytic origin of the cells if in question. Molecular studies for genetic duplications, deletions, or other alterations such as those by DNA microarray, comparative genomic hybridization (CGH), or fluorescence in situ hybridization (FISH) are currently research tools that may help distinguish benign from malignant proliferations. Loss of chromosome 7 is typical for benign nodular proliferations within CMN, whereas loss of chromosomes 9 and 10 is typical of melanoma.[22]

Melanoma has more chromosomal aberrations than congenital nevi.

Initiating Surgical Treatment and Alternative Treatments

Prophylactic excision generally begins at the age of 6 to 9 months of life, when anesthesia is safer and before the risk for transformation into melanoma has passed. In highly suspicious lesions, surgical biopsy should not be delayed. Complete surgical removal of a small congenital nevus can usually be achieved via inclusion of a 3–4 mm clinical margin of normal-appearing skin surrounding the lesion down to a level within the subcutaneous fat. Primary closure is usually attainable. The only acceptable treatment for giant CMN is surgical excision because it attempts to remove all of the lesion. Surgical removal down to the fascial plane is the treatment of choice for these large lesions. Serial excisions, tissue expanders, and skin flaps are commonly used methods for removal of larger lesions.[92-96] Other surgical techniques that aim to remove the lesion completely can be helpful.[97-99]

Because CMNs are infiltrative into the skin and tend to fill in the first few years of life, it should be recognized that surgery before the age of 2 can result in a scar with nevus surrounding it. Even if no clinically apparent nevus is present after removal, yearly follow-up is indicated in larger lesions, as melanoma has occurred 20 and 40 years after prophylactic removal of a larger CMN.

Laser, curettage, and dermabrasion have been used as partial treatments for improving the cosmetic appearance of CMN.[100,101] There is a small portion of the nevus that is removed (superficial portion) within the lesion during these procedures, leaving the deeper infiltrate of melanocytes. Because the superficial portion of the lesion is frequently the first site of change indicating malignancy, removal precludes the most common method of monitoring for malignancy. Development of melanoma 20 years after partial removal by dermabrasion has been reported.[61]

Problems associated with these alternative approaches include, in addition to incomplete removal of the lesions, scarring and recurrence of the lesion. Recurrence of the lesion with these partial treatment methods sometimes occurs as soon as within 1 year. Additional difficulty comes from the fact that recurrence of the lesion (recurrent nevus) is frequently difficult to distinguish from melanoma on biopsy.

Sun Precautions

Even in patients in whom removal of the congenital nevus has been performed, appropriate sun precautions against skin cancer and melanoma should be taught to the family including avoiding sunburn and excessive midday sun and instead seeking shade, proper application of sunscreens, and use of long-lasting broad-spectrum sunscreens. Sunburns increase the risk for developing melanoma in nevi. Broad-spectrum sunblocks that block both UVA and UVB rays are recommended. Photoprotective clothing can be a practical alternative. Patients following sun protective measures should take vitamin D3 supplements because the largest source of vitamin D synthesis comes from the influence of the sun on the skin instead of via dietary means.[102]

MELANOMA IN CHILDHOOD
Pathways to Melanoma

Differences between childhood and adult melanoma suggest that the pathophysiology of melanoma arising in congenital nevi is distinct from that of melanoma arising de novo or from an acquired nevus. The presence of a preexisting nevus in melanoma is more common in children than in adults.[103] Thirty-three percent of childhood melanoma arises in a preexisting congenital nevus.[104]

Spitzoid melanoma is also more common in children than adults, whereas lentigo maligna melanoma is much less common in children than adults. Melanoma can arise from transplacental metastasis from a melanoma in the mother (very rare), or can arise as congenital melanoma de novo in the fetus (rare). Childhood melanoma more often has atypical clinical features (nodularity and lack of pigment) for a nevus.[105] Melanoma in children most likely results from multiple pathways.[106-108]

Melanoma in young children behaves differently from melanoma in older children (young adults). There is some preliminary data to suggest that in contrast with adult melanoma, melanoma in children is more directly related to genetic instability and tendency than to ultraviolet exposure.[109] Overall for childhood melanoma, risk factors appear to be the same as in adult melanoma.[110]

Prognosis

Melanoma in childhood has a similar prognosis as in adults for a given stage. Unfortunately, children often present at a later stage.[111]

Misdiagnosis results from atypical appearance of melanoma from adults, lack of suspicion for melanoma in the young age group, delayed biopsy related to avoiding family and patient anxiety and anesthetic concerns,[73,112] and difficulty in distinguishing malignant lesions on histology of childhood lesions, such as congenital nevi and Spitz nevi.

Although some have suggested favorable prognosis for melanoma in children, when disease-specific and cause-specific deaths are compared for a given depth (correlates with American Joint Committee on Cancer [AJCC] stage), prognosis for childhood and adult melanoma is similar.[113] Just as in adult melanoma, the prognosis of childhood melanoma is related to AJCC stage at presentation[111]; yet, trends in survival of pediatric melanoma are favorable.[105,114]

Melanoma should be treated as aggressively as in adults because of the potential for equally devastating consequences.[115] Treatments are similar to those recommended for adults. Primary CNS melanoma has a uniformly poor prognosis.

Clinical Signs of Melanoma

Childhood melanoma is very rare (300–400 cases/year). Partly because of its rarity, less information is known about melanoma occurring in children. One-third of all prepubertal melanomas arise in congenital nevi. Melanoma may clinically present as a change in color at the edge of a lesion (most common presentation for smaller CMN lesions) or as a papule or nodule within the lesion (most common for large CMNs). The changes may occur rapidly or develop slowly over time. They may be obvious or subtle. It is important to recognize that in children melanoma may also present clinically as an amelanotic lesion (lesion without brown coloration) such as a red papule. Melanoma in children is more frequently associated with symptoms such as growth, pruritus, bleeding, or pain than in adults. Other signs of melanoma include asymmetric change in pigmentation (color or pattern) anywhere within a lesion, rapid growth (out of proportion to growth of the child) of a lesion, pruritus, bleeding, and pain. Any of these symptoms lasting longer than 2 weeks raises the suspicion. Pain or bleeding may occur once from trauma, but should not be repetitive. New nevi in children are not considered in and of themselves to be suspicious for melanoma, as the natural history of nevi is that they are typically acquired at a rate of 1 to 2 new nevi each year of life until middle age. In large CMNs, is it worth noting that a bleeding nodule at birth is not always melanoma, nor is a rapidly growing nodule within a CMN in an infant, as similar presentations have resulted from benign proliferative nodules. Expert dermatopathology opinion is warranted of biopsy specimens in these challenging clinical situations.

Incidence of Childhood Melanoma on the Rise

Similar to adult melanoma, childhood melanoma rates seem to be increasing, predominantly in older adolescents. Explanations may include increase in susceptibility genes, inclusion of severely atypical Spitz nevi, or increase in UV exposure and UV rates.

SUMMARY

Small congenital melanocytic nevi are most often benign in small children. Close observation over a lifetime is required because of the risk for development of melanoma. Large or giant lesions are at greatest risk for melanoma development. Larger lesions develop melanoma at an earlier age than smaller lesions and the melanoma presents at deeper layers in the skin. Patients with large CMN in a posterior axial location or with multiple satellite lesions are at risk for the development of neurocutaneous melanosis. Benign congenital nevi can become symptomatic with irritative symptoms or change in a lesion indicating the need for biopsy. When treatment is considered, surgical removal is still considered the best approach; however, special circumstances may warrant use of an alternative method for treatment.

It should be kept in mind that removal of a congenital nevus does not remove the risk of melanoma completely because melanoma more frequently arises in noncongenital nevus sites on the skin. Patients should be counseled on the signs and symptoms of melanoma and appropriate sun precautions.

REFERENCES

1. Aguilera P, Puig S, Guilabert A, et al. Prevalence study of nevi in children from Barcelona. Dermoscopy, constitutional and environmental factors. Dermatology 2009;218(3):203–14.
2. Chatproedprai S, Wananukul S. Survey of common cutaneous lesions in healthy infants at the well baby clinic. J Med Assoc Thai 2008;91(9):1356–9.
3. McLean DI, Gallagher RP. "Sunburn" freckles, cafe-au-lait macules, and other pigmented lesions of schoolchildren: the Vancouver Mole Study. J Am Acad Dermatol 1995;32(4):565–70.
4. Rivers JK, MacLennan R, Kelly JW, et al. The eastern Australian childhood nevus study: prevalence of atypical nevi, congenital nevus-like nevi, and other pigmented lesions. J Am Acad Dermatol 1995;32(6):957–63.
5. Yucesan S, Dindar H, Olcay I, et al. Prevalence of congenital abnormalities in Turkish school children. Eur J Epidemiol 1993;9(4):373–80.
6. Rhodes AR, Slifman NR, Korf BR. Familial aggregation of small congenital nevomelanocytic nevi. Am J Med Genet 1985;22(2):315–26.
7. Kopf AW, Bart RS, Hennessey P. Congenital nevocytic nevi and malignant melanomas. J Am Acad Dermatol 1979;1(2):123–30.
8. Lorentzen M, Pers M, Bretteville-Jensen G. The incidence of malignant transformation in giant pigmented nevi. Scand J Plast Reconstr Surg 1977;11(2):163–7.
9. Rhodes AR, Sober AJ, Day CL, et al. The malignant potential of small congenital nevocellular nevi. An estimate of association based on a histologic study of 234 primary cutaneous melanomas. J Am Acad Dermatol 1982;6(2):230–41.
10. Rhodes AR, Weinstock MA, Fitzpatrick TB, et al. Risk factors for cutaneous melanoma. A practical method of recognizing predisposed individuals. JAMA 1987;258(21):3146–54.
11. Lanier VC Jr, Pickrell KL, Georgiade NG. Congenital giant nevi: clinical and pathological considerations. Plast Reconstr Surg 1976;58(1):48–54.
12. Marghoob AA, Borrego JP, Halpern AC. Congenital melanocytic nevi: treatment modalities and management options. Semin Cutan Med Surg 2007;26(4): 231–40.
13. Makkar HS, Frieden IJ. Congenital melanocytic nevi: an update for the pediatrician. Curr Opin Pediatr 2002;14(4):397–403.
14. Rhodes AR, Albert LS, Weinstock MA. Congenital nevomelanocytic nevi: proportionate area expansion during infancy and early childhood. J Am Acad Dermatol 1996;34(1):51–62.

15. Ruiz-Maldonado R. Measuring congenital melanocytic nevi. Pediatr Dermatol 2004;21(2):178–9.
16. Schaffer JV, Orlow SJ, Lazova R, et al. Speckled lentiginous nevus: within the spectrum of congenital melanocytic nevi. Arch Dermatol 2001;137(2):172–8.
17. Vidaurri-de la CH, Happle R. Two distinct types of speckled lentiginous nevi characterized by macular versus papular speckles. Dermatology 2006;212(1): 53–8.
18. Stefanaki C, Antoniou C, Stefanaki K, et al. Bcl-2 and Bax in congenital naevi. Br J Dermatol 2006;154(6):1175–9.
19. Takayama H, Nagashima Y, Hara M, et al. Immunohistochemical detection of the c-met proto-oncogene product in the congenital melanocytic nevus of an infant with neurocutaneous melanosis. J Am Acad Dermatol 2001;44(3):538–40.
20. Heimann P, Ogur G, De Busscher C, et al. Chromosomal findings in cultured melanocytes from a giant congenital nevus. Cancer Genet Cytogenet 1993; 68(1):74–7.
21. Dopp E, Papp T, Schiffmann D. Detection of hyperdiploidy and chromosome breakage affecting the 1 (1cen-q12) region in lentigo malignant melanoma (LMM), superficial spreading melanoma (SSM) and congenital nevus (CN) cells in vitro by the multicolor FISH technique. Cancer Lett 1997;120(2):157–63.
22. Bastian BC, Xiong J, Frieden IJ, et al. Genetic changes in neoplasms arising in congenital melanocytic nevi: differences between nodular proliferations and melanomas. Am J Pathol 2002;161(4):1163–9.
23. Droitcourt C, Adenis-Lamarre E, Ezzedine K, et al. Blaschkolinear congenital melanocytic nevus. Dermatology 2009;219(2):182–3.
24. Torrelo A, Baselga E, Nagore E, et al. Delineation of the various shapes and patterns of nevi. Eur J Dermatol 2005;15(6):439–50.
25. Boente Mdel C, Asial RA. Desmoplastic hairless hypopigmented nevus (DHHN). A distinct variant of giant melanocytic nevus. Eur J Dermatol 2005;15(6):451–3.
26. Wu JJ, Markus RF, Orengo IF. Nonpigmented nodule on the shoulder: amelanotic congenital nevus. Int J Dermatol 2004;43(4):312.
27. Guerra-Tapia A, Isarria MJ. Periocular vitiligo with onset around a congenital divided nevus of the eyelid. Pediatr Dermatol 2005;22(5):427–9.
28. Itin PH, Lautenschlager S. Acquired leukoderma in congenital pigmented nevus associated with vitiligo-like depigmentation. Pediatr Dermatol 2002;19(1):73–5.
29. Kerr OA, Schofield O. Halo congenital nevus. Pediatr Dermatol 2003;20(6): 541–2.
30. Martin JM, Jorda E, Monteagudo C, et al. Desmoplastic giant congenital nevus with progressive depigmentation. J Am Acad Dermatol 2007;56(Suppl 2): S10–4.
31. Tokura Y, Yamanaka K, Wakita H, et al. Halo congenital nevus undergoing spontaneous regression. Involvement of T-cell immunity in involution and presence of circulating anti-nevus cell IgM antibodies. Arch Dermatol 1994;130(8):1036–41.
32. Leung AK, Kao CP, Robson WL. A giant congenital nevus spilus in an 8-year-old girl. Adv Ther 2006;23(5):701–4.
33. Yoneyama K, Kamada N, Mizoguchi M, et al. Malignant melanoma and acquired dermal melanocytosis on congenital nevus spilus. J Dermatol 2005;32(6):454–8.
34. Rose C, Kaddu S, El-Sherif TF, et al. A distinctive type of widespread congenital melanocytic nevus with large nodules. J Am Acad Dermatol 2003;49(4):732–5.
35. Tosti A, Baran R, Piraccini BM, et al. Nail matrix nevi: a clinical and histopathologic study of twenty-two patients. J Am Acad Dermatol 1996;34(5 Pt 1):765–71.

36. Borbujo J, Jara M, Cortes L, et al. A newborn with nodular ulcerated lesion on a giant congenital nevus. Pediatr Dermatol 2000;17(4):299–301.
37. Precursors to malignant melanoma. National Institutes of Health Consensus Development Conference Statement, 1983. J Am Acad Dermatol 1984;10(4): 683–8.
38. Ackerman AB. A mistake I made from which I learned much: melanoma in a pre-existing congenital nevus of Unna's type. Int J Surg Pathol 2003;11(3):213–7.
39. Hoang MP, Rakheja D, Amirkhan RH. Rosette formation within a proliferative nodule of an atypical combined melanocytic nevus in an adult. Am J Dermatopathol 2003;25(1):35–9.
40. Groben PA, Harvell JD, White WL. Epithelioid blue nevus: neoplasm Sui generis or variation on a theme? Am J Dermatopathol 2000;22(6):473–88.
41. Reed RJ. Giant congenital nevi: a conceptualization of patterns. J Invest Dermatol 1993;100(3):300S–12S.
42. Sowa J, Kobayashi H, Ishii M, et al. Histopathologic findings in Unna's nevus suggest it is a tardive congenital nevus. Am J Dermatopathol 2008;30(6): 561–6.
43. Carroll CB, Ceballos P, Perry AE, et al. Severely atypical medium-sized congenital nevus with widespread satellitosis and placental deposits in a neonate: the problem of congenital melanoma and its simulants. J Am Acad Dermatol 1994; 30(5 Pt 2):825–8.
44. van Dijk MC, Aben KK, van Hees F, et al. Expert review remains important in the histopathological diagnosis of cutaneous melanocytic lesions. Histopathology 2008;52(2):139–46.
45. Fernandez-Guarino M, Boixeda P, de Las Heras E, et al. Phakomatosis pigmentovascularis: clinical findings in 15 patients and review of the literature. J Am Acad Dermatol 2008;58(1):88–93.
46. Langenbach N, Hohenleutner U, Landthaler M. Phacomatosis pigmentokeratotica: speckled-lentiginous nevus in association with nevus sebaceus. Dermatology 1998;197(4):377–80.
47. Matsui T, Kageshita T, Ishihara T, et al. Hypercalcemia in a patient with malignant melanoma arising in congenital giant pigmented nevus. A case of increased serum level of parathyroid hormone-related protein. Dermatology 1998;197(1): 65–8.
48. Pattee SF, Hansen RC, Bangert JL, et al. Giant congenital nevus with progressive sclerodermoid reaction in a newborn. Pediatr Dermatol 2001; 18(4):320–4.
49. Weinberg JM, Schutzer PJ, Harris RM, et al. Melanoma arising in nevus spilus. Cutis 1998;61(5):287–9.
50. Rhodes AR, Silverman RA, Harrist TJ, et al. Mucocutaneous lentigines, cardiomucocutaneous myxomas, and multiple blue nevi: the "LAMB" syndrome. J Am Acad Dermatol 1984;10(1):72–82.
51. Hoang MP, Sinkre P, Albores-Saavedra J. Rhabdomyosarcoma arising in a congenital melanocytic nevus. Am J Dermatopathol 2002;24(1):26–9.
52. Amagai N, Williams CM. Malignant melanoma arising from a small congenital nevus in a black child. Arch Dermatol 1993;129(9):1215–7.
53. Betti R, Inselvini E, Vergani R, et al. Small congenital nevi associated with melanoma: case reports and considerations. J Dermatol 2000;27(9):583–90.
54. Crowson AN, Magro CM, Sanchez-Carpintero I, et al. The precursors of malignant melanoma. Recent Results Cancer Res 2002;160:75–84.

55. Bouffard D, Barnhill RL, Mihm MC, et al. Very late metastasis (27 years) of cutaneous malignant melanoma arising in a halo giant congenital nevus. Dermatology 1994;189(2):162–6.
56. Berwick M, Wiggins C. The current epidemiology of cutaneous malignant melanoma. Front Biosci 2006;11:1244–54.
57. Hu W, Nelson JE, Mohney CA, et al. Malignant melanoma arising in a pregnant African American woman with a congenital blue nevus. Dermatol Surg 2004; 30(12 Pt 2):1530–2.
58. Doherty SD, George S, Prieto VG, et al. Segmental neurofibromatosis in association with a large congenital nevus and malignant melanoma. Dermatol Online J 2006;12(7):22.
59. Miard F, Watier E, Pailheret JP, et al. [Malignant melanoma in a 7-year-old child. A report of a dramatic case]. Ann Chir Plast Esthet 1997;42(4):338–42 [in French].
60. Zeren-Bilgin I, Gur S, Aydin O, et al. Melanoma arising in a hairy nevus spilus. Int J Dermatol 2006;45(11):1362–4.
61. Zutt M, Kretschmer L, Emmert S, et al. Multicentric malignant melanoma in a giant melanocytic congenital nevus 20 years after dermabrasion in adulthood. Dermatol Surg 2003;29(1):99–101.
62. Swerdlow AJ, English JS, Qiao Z. The risk of melanoma in patients with congenital nevi: a cohort study. J Am Acad Dermatol 1995;32(4):595–9.
63. Elder DE. The blind men and the elephant. Different views of small congenital nevi. Arch Dermatol 1985;121(10):1263–5.
64. Rhodes AR, Melski JW. Small congenital nevocellular nevi and the risk of cutaneous melanoma. J Pediatr 1982;100(2):219–24.
65. Sober AJ, Burstein JM. Precursors to skin cancer. Cancer 1995;75(Suppl 2): 645–50.
66. Kaplan EN. Malignant potential of large congenital nevi. West J Med 1974; 121(3):226.
67. Rhodes AR, Wood WC, Sober AJ, et al. Nonepidermal origin of malignant melanoma associated with a giant congenital nevocellular nevus. Plast Reconstr Surg 1981;67(6):782–90.
68. Ruiz-Maldonado R, del Rosario Barona-Mazuera M, Hidalgo-Galvan LR, et al. Giant congenital melanocytic nevi, neurocutaneous melanosis and neurological alterations. Dermatology 1997;195(2):125–8.
69. Marghoob AA, Agero AL, Benvenuto-Andrade C, et al. Large congenital melanocytic nevi, risk of cutaneous melanoma, and prophylactic surgery. J Am Acad Dermatol 2006;54(5):868–70.
70. Quaba AA, Wallace AF. The incidence of malignant melanoma (0 to 15 years of age) arising in "large" congenital nevocellular nevi. Plast Reconstr Surg 1986; 78(2):174–81.
71. Tannous ZS, Mihm MC Jr, Sober AJ, et al. Congenital melanocytic nevi: clinical and histopathologic features, risk of melanoma, and clinical management. J Am Acad Dermatol 2005;52(2):197–203.
72. Mehregan AH, Mehregan DA. Malignant melanoma in childhood. Cancer 1993; 71(12):4096–103.
73. Jafarian F, Powell J, Kokta V, et al. Malignant melanoma in childhood and adolescence: report of 13 cases. J Am Acad Dermatol 2005;53(5):816–22.
74. Zaal LH, Mooi WJ, Klip H, et al. Risk of malignant transformation of congenital melanocytic nevi: a retrospective nationwide study from The Netherlands. Plast Reconstr Surg 2005;116(7):1902–9.

75. Berg P, Lindelof B. Congenital melanocytic naevi and cutaneous melanoma. Melanoma Res 2003;13(5):441–5.
76. Menon K, Dusza SW, Marghoob AA, et al. Classification and prevalence of pigmented lesions in patients with total-body photographs at high risk of developing melanoma. J Cutan Med Surg 2006;10(2):85–91.
77. Adler N, Dorafshar AH, Bauer BS, et al. Tissue expander infections in pediatric patients: management and outcomes. Plast Reconstr Surg 2009;124(2): 484–9.
78. Fox H. Neurocutaneous melanocytosis. In: Vinken PJ, Bruyn GW, editors. Handbook of clinical neurology. Amsterdam (The Netherlands): North-Holland; 1972. p. 414–28.
79. Kadonaga JN, Frieden IJ. Neurocutaneous melanosis: definition and review of the literature. J Am Acad Dermatol 1991;24(5 Pt 1):747–55.
80. DeDavid M, Orlow SJ, Provost N, et al. Neurocutaneous melanosis: clinical features of large congenital melanocytic nevi in patients with manifest central nervous system melanosis. J Am Acad Dermatol 1996;35(4):529–38.
81. Foster RD, Williams ML, Barkovich AJ, et al. Giant congenital melanocytic nevi: the significance of neurocutaneous melanosis in neurologically asymptomatic children. Plast Reconstr Surg 2001;107(4):933–41.
82. Frieden IJ, Williams ML, Barkovich AJ. Giant congenital melanocytic nevi: brain magnetic resonance findings in neurologically asymptomatic children. J Am Acad Dermatol 1994;31(3 Pt 1):423–9.
83. Kadonaga JN, Barkovich AJ, Edwards MS, et al. Neurocutaneous melanosis in association with the Dandy-Walker complex. Pediatr Dermatol 1992;9(1):37–43.
84. Agero AL, Benvenuto-Andrade C, Dusza SW, et al. Asymptomatic neurocutaneous melanocytosis in patients with large congenital melanocytic nevi: a study of cases from an Internet-based registry. J Am Acad Dermatol 2005;53(6):959–65.
85. Fishman C, Mihm MC Jr, Sober AJ. Diagnosis and management of nevi and cutaneous melanoma in infants and children. Clin Dermatol 2002;20(1):44–50.
86. Lawrence CM. Treatment options for giant congenital naevi. Clin Exp Dermatol 2000;25(1):7–11.
87. Zangari A, Bernardini ML, Tallarico R, et al. Indications for excision of nevi and melanoma diagnosed in a pediatric surgical unit. J Pediatr Surg 2007;42(8): 1412–6.
88. Pearson GD, Goodman M, Sadove AM. Congenital nevus: the Indiana University's approach to treatment. J Craniofac Surg 2005;16(5):915–20.
89. Garrido-Rios AA, Carrera C, Puig S, et al. Homogeneous blue pattern in an acral congenital melanocytic nevus. Dermatology 2008;217(4):315–7.
90. Changchien L, Dusza SW, Agero AL, et al. Age- and site-specific variation in the dermoscopic patterns of congenital melanocytic nevi: an aid to accurate classification and assessment of melanocytic nevi. Arch Dermatol 2007;143(8): 1007–14.
91. Cribier BJ, Santinelli F, Grosshans E. Lack of clinical-pathological correlation in the diagnosis of congenital naevi. Br J Dermatol 1999;141(6):1004–9.
92. Fujiwara M, Nakamura Y, Fukamizu H. Treatment of giant congenital nevus of the back by convergent serial excision. J Dermatol 2008;35(9):608–10.
93. Hurvitz KA, Rosen H, Meara JG. Pediatric cervicofacial tissue expansion. Int J Pediatr Otorhinolaryngol 2005;69(11):1509–13.
94. Gosain AK, Santoro TD, Larson DL, et al. Giant congenital nevi: a 20-year experience and an algorithm for their management. Plast Reconstr Surg 2001;108(3): 622–36.

95. Kruk-Jeromin J, Lewandowicz E, Rykala J. Surgical treatment of pigmented melanocytic nevi depending upon their size and location. Acta Chir Plast 1999; 41(1):20–4.

96. Landau AG, Hudson DA, Adams K, et al. Full-thickness skin grafts: maximizing graft take using negative pressure dressings to prepare the graft bed. Ann Plast Surg 2008;60(6):661–6.

97. Donelan MB, Garcia JA. Purse-string closure of scalp defects following tissue expansion: an effective aesthetic alternative. J Plast Reconstr Aesthet Surg 2008;61(4):419–22.

98. Earle SA, Marshall DM. Management of giant congenital nevi with artificial skin substitutes in children. J Craniofac Surg 2005;16(5):904–7.

99. Thomas WO, Rayburn S, LeBlanc RT, et al. Artificial skin in the treatment of a large congenital nevus. South Med J 2001;94(3):325–8.

100. Michel JL, Caillet-Chomel L. [Treatment of giant congenital nevus with high-energy pulsed CO2 laser]. Arch Pediatr 2001;8(11):1185–94 [in French].

101. Rompel R, Moser M, Petres J. Dermabrasion of congenital nevocellular nevi: experience in 215 patients. Dermatology 1997;194(3):261–7.

102. Reichrath J. Skin cancer prevention and UV-protection: how to avoid vitamin D-deficiency? Br J Dermatol 2009;161(Suppl 3):54–60.

103. Scalzo DA, Hida CA, Toth G, et al. Childhood melanoma: a clinicopathological study of 22 cases. Melanoma Res 1997;7(1):63–8.

104. Ceballos PI, Ruiz-Maldonado R, Mihm MC Jr. Melanoma in children. N Engl J Med 1995;332(10):656–62.

105. Ferrari A, Bono A, Baldi M, et al. Does melanoma behave differently in younger children than in adults? A retrospective study of 33 cases of childhood melanoma from a single institution. Pediatrics 2005;115(3):649–54.

106. Barnhill RL. Childhood melanoma. Semin Diagn Pathol 1998;15(3):189–94.

107. Prosdocimo T, Smith M, Polack EP. The diagnosis and treatment of childhood melanoma. W V Med J 2002;98(4):149–51.

108. Schaffer JV. Pigmented lesions in children: when to worry. Curr Opin Pediatr 2007;19(4):430–40.

109. Uribe P, Wistuba II, Solar A, et al. Comparative analysis of loss of heterozygosity and microsatellite instability in adult and pediatric melanoma. Am J Dermatopathol 2005;27(4):279–85.

110. Whiteman DC, Valery P, McWhirter W, et al. Risk factors for childhood melanoma in Queensland, Australia. Int J Cancer 1997;70(1):26–31.

111. Saenz NC, Saenz-Badillos J, Busam K, et al. Childhood melanoma survival. Cancer 1999;85(3):750–4.

112. Jafari M, Papp T, Kirchner S, et al. Analysis of ras mutations in human melanocytic lesions: activation of the ras gene seems to be associated with the nodular type of human malignant melanoma. J Cancer Res Clin Oncol 1995;121(1):23–30.

113. Livestro DP, Kaine EM, Michaelson JS, et al. Melanoma in the young: differences and similarities with adult melanoma: a case-matched controlled analysis. Cancer 2007;110(3):614–24.

114. Lewis KG. Trends in pediatric melanoma mortality in the United States, 1968 through 2004. Dermatol Surg 2008;34(2):152–9.

115. Huynh PM, Grant-Kels JM, Grin CM. Childhood melanoma: update and treatment. Int J Dermatol 2005;44(9):715–23.

Epidermal Nevi

Heather A. Brandling-Bennett, MD[a], Kimberly D. Morel, MD[b],*

> **KEYWORDS**
> • Nevi • Keratinocytes • Epidermal cells • Nevus sebaceous

Nevi or nests of cells may be made up of a variety of cell types. The cell types that live in the epidermis include epidermal cells or keratinocytes, sebaceous glands, hair follicles, apocrine and eccrine glands, and smooth muscle cells. This article discusses epidermal or keratinocyte nevi, nevus sebaceous, nevus comedonicus, smooth muscle hamartomas and inflammatory linear verrucous epidermal nevi. Syndromes associated with epidermal nevi are also reviewed.

EPIDERMAL NEVI

Epidermal nevi are noted at birth or within the first year as a linear tan patch or thin plaque. The linear pattern often follows Blaschko lines, which are believed to represent patterns of epidermal migration during embryogenesis (**Figs. 1** and **2**). Rarely, epidermal nevi do not develop until later in childhood. Initially, they may present as flat tan soft or velvety plaques. The natural history of epidermal nevi is that, around the time of puberty, they tend to become thicker, verrucous, and hyperpigmented.[1]

Although epidermal nevi may affect some of the population as an isolated finding, they may occur in association with certain syndromes or represent mosaic forms of genetically inherited conditions. Therefore, the clinician must be cognizant of the associated syndromes and conditions when presented with a patient with an epidermal nevus.[2,3] The finding of an epidermal nevus warrants a full physical examination to evaluate for other features that may been seen in association with epidermal nevi, such as Proteus syndrome and others that are described in more detail in this article. Rarely, extensive epidermal nevi may present with extensive cutaneous involvement alone. The terms that may be seen in the literature to describe the presentation of extensive epidermal nevi are systematized epidermal nevus or nevus unius lateralis.

Histologically, epidermal nevi reveal hyperkeratosis and papillomatosis. The microscopic findings are the same as seen in seborrheic keratoses, therefore the specimen must be labeled with the clinical suspicion or the morphologic features of the plaque noted in order for the histopathologist to render a clinically relevant diagnosis.

---

[a] University of Washington, Seattle Children's Hospital, 4800 Sand Point Way NE, Seattle, WA 98105, USA
[b] Department of Dermatology, Morgan Stanley Children's Hospital of New York Presbyterian, Columbia University, 161 Fort Washington Avenue, New York, NY 10032, USA
* Corresponding author.
E-mail address: km208@columbia.edu

Pediatr Clin N Am 57 (2010) 1177–1198
doi:10.1016/j.pcl.2010.07.004
0031-3955/10/$ – see front matter © 2010 Elsevier Inc. All rights reserved.

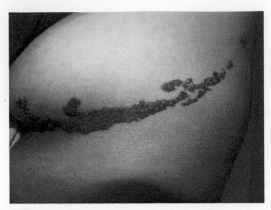

Fig. 1. Linear epidermal nevus following the lines of Blaschko.

Thirty-three percent of epidermal nevi of keratinocyte differentiation have been found to have a mutation in the fibroblast growth factor receptor 3 (FGFR3) gene. Acquired seborrheic keratoses have also been found to have a mutation in the FGFR3 receptor.[4–6] It is also important to distinguish the histologic features of epidermolytic hyperkeratosis (EHK). EHK is associated with mutations in the keratin gene. Patients with cutaneous epidermal nevi revealing EHK histology may transmit this gene to their offspring with widespread cutaneous involvement, as discussed later in this article.[7] The potential for malignant transformation of epidermal nevi is low,[8,9] but is higher in certain subtypes of nevi, such as nevus sebaceous.

Treatment of epidermal nevi may be difficult. Topical therapies such as off-label use of topical retinoids, and destructive modalities such as electrodessication or cryotherapy may temporally improve the appearance of the lesion, but recurrence is the rule. Definitive treatment involves full-thickness excision, which may not be possible in large or extensive lesions. Carbon dioxide laser is an alternative option; however, scarring and pigmentary alteration are potential permanent complications, especially in patients with darker skin types.[10,11]

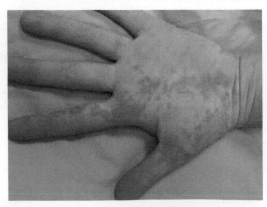

Fig. 2. Linear epidermal nevus with palmar involvement.

NEVUS SEBACEOUS

Nevus sebaceous, also referred to as nevus sebaceus of Jadassohn, is a common hamartoma of the epidermis, hair follicles and sebaceous and apocrine glands. Nevus sebaceous usually presents at birth as a yellow-orange to pink, finely papillomatous, alopecic plaque that is often oval or linear (**Fig. 3**). The size may vary from less than a centimeter to several centimeters in length, and a patient can rarely have multiple lesions. There are a few reports of unusually large and exophytic lesions for which histopathology was consistent with nevus sebaceous.[12,13] There is a predilection for the scalp, but the next most common location is the face, and they may also occur on the neck, trunk, or, rarely, elsewhere on the body.[14–16] These lesions generally grow proportionately with the child. During puberty, they have a tendency to become more raised, verrucous, and greasy, at least in part because of androgen stimulation of sebaceous glands.[17,18]

There is debate about the risk of developing benign and malignant tumors within nevus sebaceous. Because studies are based on retrospective slide reviews of excised lesions, the true incidence and lifetime risk of malignancy is unknown. Early reports suggested a high rate of developing basal cell carcinomas.[19,20] More recent studies have suggested that trichoblastoma and syringocystadenoma papilliferum are the most common neoplasms to develop in nevus sebaceous, usually in adulthood.[14,15,21] Several retrospective slide reviews of a series of excised lesions found

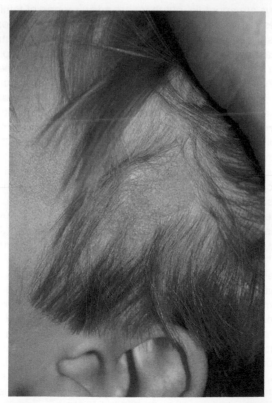

Fig. 3. Nevus sebaceous.

malignant neoplasms in 0% to 2.7% of cases.[14–16,21–23] Jaqueti and colleagues[14] reviewed previously published reports and concluded that many of the neoplasms previously diagnosed as basal cell carcinomas would have been better interpreted as trichoblastomas or primitive follicular induction. Multiple other benign neoplasms have been reported to arise in nevus sebaceous, including viral warts, sebaceoma, trichilemmoma, apocrine hidrocystoma or cystadenoma, keratoacanthoma, seborrheic keratosis and melanocytic nevus.[14,15,21]

There are reports of more unusual or aggressive malignant neoplasms arising in adults with nevus sebaceous, including squamous cell carcinoma,[20,24] apocrine carcinoma,[20] sebaceous carcinoma,[25–27] eccrine porocarcinoma,[28] adenocarcinoma[29] and mucoepidermoid (adenosquamous) carcinoma.[30]

There are a few retrospective studies specifically about nevus sebaceous in children. Barkham and colleagues[31] reviewed 63 cases of nevus sebaceous evaluated at a children's hospital, of which 50% were excised, none of which had malignant change, only 1 had a benign neoplasm. Cribier and colleagues[15] reported benign neoplasms in 1.9% of lesions excised from prepubertal children and 11.6% from pubertal children. Rosen and colleagues[16] reviewed 651 excised lesions in children and found that 0.8% had basal cell carcinomas (the youngest at 9.7 years of age), and 2.2% had benign neoplasms. There are a few additional reports of basal cell carcinoma developing in nevus sebaceous in children less than 16 years of age.[32] There are rare reports of squamous cell carcinomas arising within nevus sebaceous in an 11 year old and a 15 year old.[33,34]

Nevus sebaceous has been theorized to arise from genetic mosaicism. Most cases of nevus sebaceous are sporadic, but there are a few reports of familial cases.[35–39] It has been hypothesized that paradominant inheritance, whereby postzygotic loss of heterozygosity results in a mosaic homozygous or hemizygous state may explain the rare familial cases of nevus sebaceous.[35,36,40] Carlson and colleagues[41] found a high prevalence (82%) of human papillomavirus (HPV) DNA in nevus sebaceous. They postulated that HPV infection of fetal epidermal stem cells could play a role in the pathogenesis of nevus sebaceous. Xin and colleagues[42] found that 8 of 20 (40%) cases of nevus sebaceous exhibited loss of heterozygosity for the human homolog of the Drosophilia patched (PTCH) gene, the tumor suppressor gene implicated in basal cell nevus syndrome. This may help explain the risk of development of basal cell carcinomas within nevus sebaceous.

Histopathology of a nevus sebaceous reveals variable epidermal hyperplasia with hyperkeratosis, acanthosis, or papillomatosis that may become more prominent in time.[14] Sebaceous glands may be hyperplastic and numerous, but may also be diminished or even absent. They may be located high in the dermis and unrelated to a hair follicle, sometimes communicating directly with the epidermis.[43] Hair follicles are usually decreased, absent, or immature. Ectopic apocrine glands may be present in the lower dermis.[14,43,44]

Removal of a nevus sebaceous is best done by surgical excision, but the necessity and timing of excision is controversial. Some investigators have argued that because the incidence of malignant neoplasms in nevus sebaceous is extremely rare, early excision is not necessary.[14,15,21,31] Other investigators have argued that prophylactic excision is still warranted because malignant transformation can occur and even benign growths often require surgical intervention.[16,45] Some patients or their families also desire excision for cosmetic concerns. Optimal timing for excision may depend on various factors, including size and location of the lesion, and the risks and benefits of general anesthesia versus local anesthesia. Local anesthesia is often being an option for less extensive lesions when the patient is older.

Carbon dioxide laser and photodynamic therapy have been used to treat nevus sebaceous for cosmetic reasons,[46,47] but these modalities do not completely remove the lesion, leaving a risk of recurrence and development of secondary neoplasms.

NEVUS COMEDONICUS

Nevus comedonicus is a developmental anomaly of the pilosebaceous unit that typically presents at birth or during childhood. Clinically, a nevus comedonicus presents as a linear array or cluster of dilated follicular orifices plugged with keratin, resembling comedones. Larger lesions typically follow Blaschko lines and extensive involvement of half the body has been described.[48,49] Nevus comedonicus seems to have a predilection for the face, neck, or trunk, but can involve the extremities, scalp, or genitalia.[48,50] Although usually unilateral, there are reports of bilateral lesions.[51,52] Inflammatory variants with pustules, cysts, secondary bacterial infections, and scarring can occur.[48,49,53] Malignant change is rare, but there are reports of basal cell carcinoma and squamous cell carcinoma arising within nevus comedonicus.[54,55]

It has been hypothesized that nevus comedonicus arises from a developmental defect in the mesodermal component of the pilosebaceous unit, where in the resulting follicular structure is only able to produce accumulating soft keratin.[56] Others have suggested that nevus comedonicus is a variant of epidermal nevus involving the hair follicle.[57] Munro and Wilkie[58] identified a somatic mutation in fibroblast growth factor receptor 2 (FGFR2), in an acneiform nevus. The severe acne found in certain patients with craniosynostosis and *FGF* mutations led to the search for the association. An immunohistochemical study found increased filaggrin, but not cytokeratin, expression in closed comedones of nevus comedonicus. Further studies are needed to elucidate the role of filaggrin in the pathogenesis of nevus comedonicus.[59]

Histopathology of nevus comedonicus reveals cystically dilated hair follicles forming epidermal invaginations filled with lamellar keratin.[50] EHK has been described in the keratinocytes of the follicular epithelial wall.[57,60] There is a report of a child with generalized EHK (also known as bullous congenital ichthyosiform erythroderma), whose father had 2 small patches of nevus comedonicus on his neck and back with biopsies from his back revealing histopathologic features of EHK within the nevus comedonicus.[61]

Cosmetically concerning or inflammatory lesions warrant treatment. Smaller, localized lesions may be excised. Larger, more extensive lesions can be challenging to treat. Potential topical therapies include ammonium lactate and other keratolytics, topical retinoids, calcipotriene, or tacalcitol.[51,52,62] Inflammatory lesions may be treated with oral antibiotics or intralesional corticosteroids.[48,53] Oral isotretinoin has limited efficacy, but may decrease formation of suppurative cystic lesions.[49] Hormonal therapy has been used with some benefit.[63] Other reported treatment options include manual extraction of keratin plugs, dermabrasion, and the erbium:yyttrium-aluminum-garnet (YAG) laser.[64] A commercially available pore strip was successfully used to remove keratin plugs in 2 patients with nevus comedonicus.[65]

BECKER NEVUS

Becker nevus, also referred to as Becker melanosis or pigmented hairy epidermal nevus, is a common type of epidermal nevus that occurs most frequently on the trunk or proximal upper extremities of young men (**Fig. 4**). Studies of young male military recruits in France and Italy found a prevalence ranging from 0.25% to 2.1%.[66–68] Many more cases have been reported in males than females, but the true male/female ratio is unknown.[69,70] Becker nevus typically presents as a hyperpigmented patch with

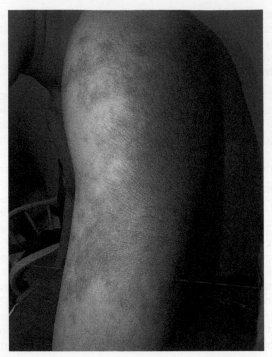

Fig. 4. Becker nevus.

irregular borders that gradually enlarges for a few years then remains stable. Hypertrichosis within the lesion is common, but not universal. It can also be associated with acneiform eruptions. A Becker nevus may become more elevated when stroked or rubbed because of piloerection, referred to as pseudo-Darier sign. Although they usually appear during adolescence, there are reports of Becker nevi occurring at birth or during early childhood.[71,72] Some congenital lesions may be better classified as congenital smooth muscle hamartomas.[2] Lesions are typically located on the trunk or proximal upper extremities, but they can occur elsewhere, including the face[73,74] and lower extremities.[75] Most are solitary and unilateral, although multiple and bilateral Becker nevi have been reported.[76–78]

There have been rare reports of familial Becker nevus.[72,79] Happle[80] and others have hypothesized that paradominant inheritance (postzygotic loss of heterozygosity occurring at an early stage of development) best explains the usually sporadic occurrence and mosaic distribution of these lesions.[81] Increased androgen receptors have been found in Becker nevi by ligand-binding assays, protein expression, and immunohistochemisty.[82–84] It has been suggested that increased sensitivity to androgens plays a role in pathogenesis of these lesions. Androgen stimulation may help explain clinical and histopathological features such as onset during puberty, hypertrichosis, acneiform eruptions, acanthosis, and dermal thickening.[83]

Histopathological findings may be subtle, with acanthosis, elongation of rete ridges, variable hyperkeratosis, and basal layer hyperpigmentation. There is no proliferation of melanocytes. The dermis may or may not contain smooth muscle hyperplasia.[85] The common dermoscopic features have been described as the presence of a network, hair follicles, and vessels, with focal, skin furrow, and perifollicular hypopigmentation.[86]

Becker nevi are not generally considered to have malignant potential. There are few isolated reports of skin cancers developing within Becker nevi, namely malignant melanoma,[87] Bowen disease,[88] and basal cell carcinoma,[89] with the small number of reports suggesting a chance association. Fehr and colleagues[87] reported 9 patients with Becker nevi who developed malignant melanoma, although only 1 occurred within the Becker nevus. The investigators suggested that patients with a Becker nevus may have a higher incidence of other pigmented lesions such as malignant melanoma, but a true association has not been established.

Some patients seeking medical attention for these lesions only require reassurance that this is a benign condition, whereas others desire treatment because of cosmetic concerns. Excision is not generally an acceptable option, and laser treatment has had variable efficacy. Various lasers have been used to lighten the pigmentation and decrease associated hypertrichosis. A comparative study suggested that 1 treatment with an erbium:YAG laser was more effective than 3 treatments with a Q-switched Nd:YAG laser.[90] Another study suggested good to excellent response in 7 of 11 patients after multiple (2–12) treatments with a long-pulse alexandrite laser.[91] Success has also been reported with multiple (5–6) fractional resurfacing treatments using the 1550-nm wavelength erbium-doped fiber laser in 2 patients.[92]

INFLAMMATORY LINEAR VERRUCOUS EPIDERMAL NEVUS

Inflammatory linear verrucous epidermal nevus (ILVEN) is a type of epidermal nevus characterized by pruritic erythematous scaly papules and plaques. They may be present at birth or develop during early childhood. The differential diagnosis includes linear psoriasis, lichen striatus, linear lichen planus, and epidermal nevus with verrucous changes. The prognosis is variable, often waxing and waning with time. Treatment options that have been described as leading to temporary improvement include topical or intralesional steroids, topical retinoids, 5-fluorouracil, calcineurin inhibitors, and calcipotriol.[93,94] Surgical options for localized lesions may be successful.[95]

POROKERATOTIC ECCRINE OSTIAL AND DERMAL DUCT NEVUS

Porokeratotic eccrine ostial and dermal duct nevus (PEODDN) is a rare malformation often classified as an eccrine hamartoma. Clinically, it presents as hyperkeratotic papules and plaques with comedo-like punctuate pits, often filled with keratin plugs. Lesions are usually in a linear pattern, most commonly located on the palms or soles. There are several cases with widespread unilateral or bilateral lesions distributed along Blaschko lines.[96–98] Although most of these lesions are present at birth, there are reports of later onset, usually in early childhood.[24,99,100]

There are reports of linear psoriasis in 2 patients with PEODDN.[101,102] Multiple squamous cell carcinomas were found in a patient with widespread PEODDN.[103] There is another report of Bowen disease arising within a PEODDN on the sole.[104] Rarely, extracutaneous abnormalities have been described in patients with PEODDN, including seizure disorder, hemiparesis, and scoliosis in one patient,[105] developmental delay with hearing loss in another patient,[98] and ipsilateral breast hypoplasia in a recent report.[97]

Histopathology reveals epidermal invagination with a parakeratotic column resembling a cornoid lamella, overlying a dilated eccrine acrosyringium and dermal duct.[106,107] Immunohistochemical staining for carcinoembryonic antigen is positive along the cuticle of the eccrine dermal duct and acrosyringium through the channel within the parakeratotic column.[107,108]

Treatment with topical steroids, tar, phototherapy, and cryotherapy have offered little benefit.[97,106] Topical or oral retinoids have unclear efficacy.[97] Carbon dioxide laser therapy has been used successfully.[109,110] Small, localized lesions may be excised. There are isolated case reports of gradual improvement over years in patients with widespread involvement.[111,112]

SYNDROMES ASSOCIATED WITH EPIDERMAL NEVI
Epidermal Nevus Syndrome

Several syndromes may be associated with epidermal nevi. The term epidermal nevus syndrome has been used to describe the association of an epidermal nevus with systemic features potentially affecting multiple organs including neurologic, ocular, skeletal, and in rare cases, cardiac and renal anomalies.[3] Even small epidermal nevi, especially in the setting of other cutaneous findings may be associated with syndromes or warrant further consideration for neurocutaneous, genetic, or metabolic disorders such as hypophosphatemic vitamin D–resistant rickets.[113] Syndromes associated with epidermal nevi are discussed below.

Proteus Syndrome

Linear epidermal nevi are commonly found in patients with Proteus syndrome. Proteus syndrome is characterized by patchy or mosaic overgrowth of multiple tissues. The overgrowth is irregular, progressive, and usually asymmetric, most often involving a limb, but can involve any body part.[114] In addition to epidermal nevi, vascular malformations (most commonly cutaneous capillary malformations) are frequent cutaneous manifestations in Proteus syndrome. Cerebriform connective tissue nevi are less common, but fairly specific for Proteus syndrome. These are usually located on the soles of the feet and, rarely, on the hands or elsewhere, and are generally not present at birth, but evolve slowly over time. Dysregulation of fatty tissue with overgrowth and/or atrophy is often present. Several tumors have been reported in patients with Proteus syndrome, but the most specific seem to be monomorphic adenomas of the parotid glands and bilateral ovarian cystadenomas.[114,115]

The diagnosis of Proteus syndrome can be challenging and controversial. Consensus criteria for the diagnosis were proposed after a conference at the National Institutes of Health in 1998. General criteria required for diagnosis were defined as mosaic distribution of lesions, sporadic occurrence, and progressive course. To make the diagnosis, the patient then has to meet specific criteria (**Box 1**), which were later revised and clarified.[116,117] Application of these criteria to 205 cases of reported Proteus syndrome in the literature found that only 97 cases (47.3%) met diagnostic criteria, suggesting a high rate of misdiagnosis.[117] The differential diagnosis for Proteus syndrome includes neurofibromatosis type 1, Klippel-Trenaunay syndrome, hemihyperplasia and multiple lipomatosis syndrome, and other undefined overgrowth syndromes.[114,118]

The cutaneous manifestations of Proteus syndrome were reported in a cohort of 24 consecutive patients evaluated at the National Institutes of Health. The most common findings were lipomas (92%), vascular malformations (88%), plantar cerebriform connective tissue nevi (83%), epidermal nevi (67%), partial lipohypoplasia (38%), and patchy dermal hypoplasia (21%). Patients with a greater number of cutaneous abnormalities tended to have more extracutaneous abnormalities.[119]

Controversy exists regarding the genetic basis of Proteus syndrome. It has been hypothesized that the syndrome results from somatic mosaicism, with an underlying genetic mutation that would be lethal in a nonmosaic state.[115,120,121] Cowden

---

Box 1
Diagnostic criteria for Proteus syndrome

General Criteria (all 3 required for diagnosis)

  Mosaic distribution of lesions

  Sporadic occurrence

  Progressive course

Specific Criteria (either category A, or 2 from category B, or 3 from category C)

  • Cerebriform connective tissue nevus[a]

  • Linear epidermal nevus

  Asymmetric, disproportionate overgrowth of limbs, skull, external auditory canal, vertebrae, or viscera[b]

  Bilateral ovarian cystadenomas or parotid monomorphic adenoma (before second decade)

  • Dysregulated adipose tissue (unencapsulated lipomas or lipohypoplasia)

  Vascular malformations (capillary, venous, or lymphatic)

  Lung cysts

  Facial phenotype (dolichocephaly, long face, downslanting palpebral fissures, and/or minor ptosis, low nasal bridge, wide or anteverted nares, open mouth at rest)[c]

[a] Skin lesions characterized by deep grooves and gyrations.
[b] Distinguished from asymmetric, proportionate overgrowth.
[c] Facial phenotype found in patients who have mental deficiency and, in some cases, seizures and/or brain malformations.

  Adapted from Turner JT, Cohen Jr MM, Biesecker LG. Reassessment of the Proteus syndrome literature: application of diagnostic criteria to published cases. Am J Med Genet A 2004;130(2):119.

---

syndrome and Bannayan-Riley-Ruvalcaba syndrome, allelic multiple hamartoma syndromes, have been associated with autosomal dominant germline *PTEN* mutations, with a unifying designation as PTEN hamartoma tumor syndrome.[122–125] *PTEN* (phosphatase and tensin homolog) is a tumor suppressor gene that encodes a protein tyrosine phosphatase that antagonizes the phosphoinositol-3-kinase/Akt pathway. There have been reports of patients diagnosed with Proteus syndrome or Proteus-like syndrome who were found to have *PTEN* germline mutations,[126–128] which has led to debate in the literature. Some investigators have argued that the patients found to have *PTEN* mutations were likely misdiagnosed and that the use of the term Proteus-like syndrome is misleading.[129,130] There have been several series of patients with Proteus syndrome who were not found to have germline or somatic *PTEN* mutations.[119,129,131,132] Happle[133,134] suggested that cases of Proteus syndrome and Proteus-like syndrome caused by *PTEN* mutations should be more accurately categorized as a type 2 segmental manifestation of Cowden syndrome, caused by loss of the heterozygosity of the *PTEN* allele at an early stage in development. Although this debate may continue, the genetic cause in most, if not all, patients with Proteus syndrome remains unknown at this time.

Complications of Proteus syndrome include orthopedic issues from limb overgrowth, with severe functional and cosmetic consequences. Limited mobility, vascular malformations, and/or surgical intervention predispose these patients to deep venous thrombosis and pulmonary embolism, which can result in early death.[135,136]

Perioperative anticoagulant prophylaxis, but not chronic anticoagulation, has been recommended.[114] Although various tumors have been reported in patients with Proteus syndrome, there are no clear screening guidelines.[114] Evaluation of patients with suspected or confirmed Proteus syndrome should include skeletal surveys, and magnetic resonance imaging (MRI) or computed tomography (CT) imaging of the brain, chest, abdomen, and any other clinically affected areas.[115] Management of these patients requires a multidisciplinary approach, with specialty consultations as needed. The psychosocial effects of this disfiguring and debilitating condition should also be addressed.[137,138]

Linear Cowden (or PTEN) Nevus

Happle[134] proposed the terms linear Cowden nevus or linear PTEN nevus to describe a nonorganoid (ie, purely keratinocytic) epidermal nevus caused by loss of heterozygosity in a germline *PTEN* mutation. He suggested that this is a cutaneous feature of type 2 segmental Cowden syndrome (see earlier discussion), and is distinct from the epidermal nevus seen in Proteus syndrome. Happle[133,134] distinguished between the 2 types of epidermal nevi based on clinical features, describing the linear Cowden nevus as thicker and more papillomatous than the soft, velvety linear nevus seen in Proteus syndrome. However, he noted that most nonorganoid epidermal nevi are not associated with any particular syndrome.[134]

Segmental Overgrowth, Lipomatosis, Arteriovenous Malformation, and Epidermal Nevus Syndrome

Caux and colleagues[139] described 2 patients from different families who had a constellation of findings for which they proposed the acronym SOLAMEN syndrome (segmental overgrowth, lipomatosis, arteriovenous malformation, and epidermal nevus). Each of these patients had other family members who presented with classic manifestations of Cowden syndrome, and the families were found to have germline *PTEN* mutations. The 2 depicted patients had some features that were unusual for Cowden syndrome and were more reminiscent of manifestations of Proteus syndrome, including progressive overgrowth, lipomatosis, and vascular malformations, but they did not meet criteria for Proteus syndrome. The investigators suggested that the 2 proband patients had segmental exacerbation of Cowden disease. The investigators hypothesized that the findings in their 2 specified patients may be explained by germline *PTEN* mutations with mosaic inactivation of the wild-type PTEN allele resulting in homozygous loss of *PTEN* function in specific lesions. These 2 patients could also be categorized as having type 2 segmental Cowden disease as proposed by Happle.[133]

CLOVE Syndrome

Sapp and colleagues[140] delineated a syndrome of congenital lipomatous overgrowth, vascular malformations, and epidermal nevi (CLOVE syndrome) based on 7 patients who did not meet criteria for Proteus syndrome. These patients all had congenital bilateral overgrowth of the feet, and congenital, complex, truncal vascular malformations, although only 4 had linear epidermal nevi. Overgrowth in these patients was described as proportionate or ballooning, in contrast to progressive and distorting overgrowth in Proteus syndrome, with bony distortion in CLOVE syndrome only after major surgery. All 7 patients had negative *PTEN* mutation analysis. Gucev and colleagues[141] subsequently described another patient with features of CLOVE syndrome, who also had central nervous system malformations including hemimegalencephaly with agenesis of the corpus callosum; a similar case was previously reported in the literature.[142] Alomari[143,144] proposed expanding the name to CLOVES syndrome to emphasize associated scoliosis and skeletal and spinal anomalies, when he reported 18 cases characterized by truncal lipomatous masses, vascular malformations, and acral deformities. Prenatal imaging and perinatal findings of a patient with CLOVE(S) syndrome have also been reported.[145]

Nevus Sebaceous Syndrome

Almost all children with nevus sebaceous are otherwise healthy, but an association with neurologic, ocular, skeletal, or other extracutaneous manifestations defines nevus sebaceous syndrome, sometimes referred to as linear nevus sebaceous syndrome. It has also been referred to by various eponyms including Shimmelpenning syndrome, Shimmelpenning-Feuerstein-Mims syndrome, Solomon syndrome, and Jadassohn syndrome.[146] Although there are several subtypes of epidermal nevus syndromes, as discussed in this article, some cases of nevus sebaceous syndrome in the literature are simply referred to as epidermal nevus syndrome.

A review of 196 consecutive patients with nevus sebaceous found that 7% had clinical neurologic abnormalities including mental retardation and seizures, and 2% had ocular abnormalities including colobomas and choristomas.[147] Large size and centrofacial location were more common in patients with neurologic abnormalities, but 9 patients with extensive nevi and 4 patients with centrofacial nevi had no associated abnormalities. Neuroimaging was normal in 6 of 8 patients with neurologic abnormalities.[147]

The most frequent extracutaneous manifestation of nevus sebaceous syndrome is central nervous system involvement, including seizures, developmental delay, and sometimes structural brain abnormalities.[146] Ophthalmologic abnormalities are also common.[146] A range of musculoskeletal, cardiovascular, and urogenital manifestations have been described.[146,148,149] There can be associated endocrine abnormalities, including hypophosphatemic rickets and precocious puberty.[150] Intraoral lesions and neoplasm in other organs may also develop.[151]

There are several cases of aplasia cutis congenita occurring in nevus sebaceous syndrome. Happle and Konig[152] proposed the term didymosis aplasticosebacea to refer to this association. They hypothesized that it reflects twin spotting, when somatic recombination causes a heterozygous cell to give rise to 2 different homozygous daughter cells.[153,154]

Nevus sebaceous syndrome is believed to result from mosaicism of a lethal autosomal dominant gene.[70] It has been hypothesized that the timing of the mutation during embryogenesis and the resulting extent of mosaicism may determine the phenotype of patients with nevus sebaceous. A mutation occurring late in embryogenesis could result in an isolated nevus sebaceous, whereas a mutation early in embryogenesis could have more deleterious consequences manifesting as nevus sebaceous syndrome.[36] As discussed earlier, Carlson and colleagues[41] found a high incidence of HPV DNA in nevus sebaceous. They theorized that HPV infection of a pluripotent stem cell at an early stage of embryogenesis could play a role in the pathogenesis of nevus sebaceous syndrome with involvement of skin, brain, eye, and skeletal and/or other structures.

Workup for a patient with suspected nevus sebaceous syndrome should include a thorough neurologic and ophthalmogical examination, with consideration of electroencephalography, neuroimaging (CT or MRI), skeletal radiography, and analysis of liver and renal function as well as serum and urine calcium and phosphate levels.[146,155]

Phacomatosis Pigmentokeratotica

The term phacomatosis pigmentokeratotica was proposed by Happle and colleagues[156] in 1996 to refer to the association of an organoid epidermal nevus, usually with sebaceous differentiation, and a speckled-lentiginous nevus (SLN), or nevus spilus. This condition is considered by some to be one of the epidermal nevus syndromes.[2,70] Various extracutaneous abnormalities have been reported, including neurologic, ophthalmologic, musculoskeletal, and endocrine findings,[157,158] although some patients do not have extracutaneous manifestations.[159–161]

The distribution of the epidermal nevus usually follows Blaschko lines, whereas the SLN is arranged in a checkerboard pattern. The epidermal nevus and SLN can be contralateral or ipsilateral, or both can be bilateral.[158] Different types of melanocytic neoplasms can develop within the SLN, including malignant melanoma.[158,162,163] Malignancies, namely basal cell carcinomas, have been reported to develop in the nevus sebaceous.[163,164] In addition, there are a few reports of internal neoplasms in patients with phacomatosis pigmentokeratotica.[158,164,165]

Although the pathogenesis of phacomatosis pigmentokeratotica is unknown, it is hypothesized to result from twin spotting or didymosis, whereby somatic recombination during early embryogenesis causes a heterozygous stem cell to give rise to 2 different populations of daughter cells, each homozygous for a recessive mutation.[156,166]

Nevus Comedonicus Syndrome

Although often occurring in isolation, nevus comedonicus can be associated with other developmental anomalies, referred to as nevus comedonicus syndrome. Reported extracutaneous manifestations include skeletal abnormalities (scoliosis, other spinal deformities, and limb defects), ocular abnormalities (cataracts), and central nervous system abnormalities (brain dysgenesis).[167–169] Nevus comedonicus has been reported as a marker of occult spinal dysraphism.[170] Happle[70] proposed that nevus comedonicus syndrome results from mosaicism of a lethal autosomal mutation.

Becker Nevus Syndrome

Happle and Koopman[171] proposed the term Becker nevus syndrome to refer to patients with a Becker nevus and other associated developmental defects. There are multiple reports of associated ipsilateral breast hypoplasia, mainly in female patients, but also in male patients. Various musculoskeletal anomalies have been described, including scoliosis, hemivertebrae, spina bifida occulata, limb asymmetry, fused or accessory cervical ribs, pectus excavatum, pectus carinatum, bilateral internal tibial torsion, ipsilateral shoulder girdle hypoplasia, ipsilateral absence of the pectoralis major muscle, umbilical hernia, and segmental odontomaxillary dysplasia.[171–173] Associated soft tissue and cutaneous abnormalities include supernumary nipples,[174] ipsilateral patchy extramammary fatty tissue hypoplasia, hypoplasia of the contralateral labium minus, accessory scrotum, sparse hair of the ipsilateral axilla, and depression of the ipsilateral temporal region.[171,172]

Paradominant inheritance, or postzygotic loss of heterozygosity occuring at an early stage of embryogenesis resulting in mosaicism, has been proposed as the genetic basis of Becker nevus and Becker nevus syndrome. This may explain the typically sporadic occurrence as well as rare familial aggregation.[70,81,171,172,174,175]

Epidermolytic Hyperkeratosis

The clinician should also be aware that an epidermal nevus may have features of EHK, both clinically and histologically. This type of nevus represents a mosaic form of EHK. EHK is a genetic disorder of keratinization with a clinical phenotype that varies from birth to adulthood. A newborn with EHK is born with bullae and the disorder has also been known as bullous congenital ichthyosiform erythroderma (BCIE). A feature distinguishing this condition from other newborn disorders of keratinization is that the bullae may be macerated. In time, the skin becomes thickened, hence the hyperkeratosis. Older children have a palmoplantar keratoderma and may have velvety thickening of skin folds. The flexural areas are often prominently involved with thick hyperkeratotic brown scales. The genetic defect is in keratin 1 or 10. It affects approximately 1 in 300,000 individuals. Fifty percent are dominantly inherited, and 50% are sporadic or new mutations.[7,176,177]

Mosaic forms have been described in which adults may have a blaschkoiform strip of affected skin and their offspring present with full systemic findings. Adults suspected of a mosaic form of EHK should receive genetic counseling regarding the condition.[7]

For patients with epidermal nevi who have been found to be carriers of the genetic mutation for EHK, a skin biopsy of an epidermal nevus may show the histologic features of marked hyperkeratosis with lysis of the epidermal cells above the basal layer.

Ichthyosis bullosa of Siemens tends to be a milder form of EHK and may also present with epidermal-type nevi, in which the blistering occurs more superficially in the epidermal layer. The genetic defect has been described in the gene encoding K2e, which is not expressed until the mid portion of epidermal maturation.[178,179]

Congenital Hemidysplasia with Ichthyosiform Erythroderma and Limb Defects Syndrome

The cutaneous features of congenital hemidysplasia with ichthyosiform erythroderma and limb defects (CHILD) syndrome may mimic the skin lesions of inflammatory epidermal nevi. They are referred to as a unilateral ichthyosiform erythroderma, which is congenital or appears in the first few months after birth. Ptychotrophism, or the inflammatory nevi affecting intertrigineous areas, is a feature of CHILD syndrome.[180] Skeletal features and hemihypoplasia of the affected side is a feature of the syndrome. The genetic defect has been described in the NSDHL gene encoding 3β-hydrosteroid dehydrogenase.[181] There is a case of a boy with CHILD syndrome considered to be secondary to early postzygotic mosaicism.[182]

REFERENCES

1. Rogers M. Epidermal nevi and the epidermal nevus syndromes: a review of 233 cases. Pediatr Dermatol 1992;9:342–4.
2. Sugarman JL. Epidermal nevus syndromes. Semin Cutan Med Surg 2007;26: 221–30.
3. Vujevich JJ, Mancini AJ. The epidermal nevus syndromes: multisystem disorders. J Am Acad Dermatol 2004;50:957–61.
4. Hafner C, van Oers JM, Vogt T, et al. Mosaicism of activating FGFR3 mutations in human skin causes epidermal nevi. J Clin Invest 2006;116(8):2201–7.
5. Hafner C, Hartmann A, Vogt T. FGFR3 mutations in epidermal nevi and seborrheic keratoses: lessons from urothelium and skin. J Invest Dermatol 2007; 127(7):1572–3.

6. Collin B, Taylor IB, Wilkie AO, et al. Fibroblast growth factor receptor 3 (FGFR3) mutation in a verrucous epidermal naevus associated with mild facial dysmorphism. Br J Dermatol 2007;156(6):1353–6.
7. Paller AS, Syder AJ, Chan YM, et al. Genetic and clinical mosaicism in a type of epidermal nevus. N Engl J Med 1994;331(21):1408–15.
8. Hafner C, Klein A, Landthaler M, et al. Clonality of basal cell carcinoma arising in an epidermal nevus. New insights provided by molecular analysis. Dermatology 2009;218(3):278–81.
9. Hafner C, López-Knowles E, Luis NM, et al. ONCOGENIC PIK3Ca mutations occur in epidermal nevi and seborrheic keratoses with a characteristic mutation pattern. Proc Natl Acad Sci U S A 2007;104(33):13450–4.
10. Losee JE, Serletti JM, Pennino RP. Epidermal nevus syndrome: a review and case report. Ann Plast Surg 1999;43:211–4.
11. Boyce S, Alster TS. CO_2 laser treatment of epidermal nevi: long-term success. Dermatol Surg 2002;28(7):611–4.
12. Correale D, Ringpfeil F, Rogers M. Large, papillomatous, pedunculated nevus sebaceus: a new phenotype. Pediatr Dermatol 2008;25(3):355–8.
13. Saedi T, Cetas J, Chang R, et al. Newborn with sebaceous nevus of Jadassohn presenting as exophytic scalp lesion. Pediatr Neurosurg 2008;44(2):144–7.
14. Jaqueti G, Requena L, Sanchez Yus E. Trichoblastoma is the most common neoplasm developed in nevus sebaceus of Jadassohn: a clinicopathologic study of a series of 155 cases. Am J Dermatopathol 2000;22(2):108–18.
15. Cribier B, Scrivener Y, Grosshans E. Tumors arising in nevus sebaceus: a study of 596 cases. J Am Acad Dermatol 2000;42(2 Pt 1):263–8.
16. Rosen H, Schmidt B, Lam HP, et al. Management of nevus sebaceous and the risk of basal cell carcinoma: an 18-year review. Pediatr Dermatol 2009;26:676–81.
17. Person JR, Bentkover S, Longcope C. Androgen receptors are increased in nevus sebaceus. J Am Acad Dermatol 1986;15(1):120–2.
18. Hamilton KS, Johnson S, Smoller BR. The role of androgen receptors in the clinical course of nevus sebaceus of Jadassohn. Mod Pathol 2001;14(6):539–42.
19. Mehregan AH, Pinkus H. Life history of organoid nevi. special reference to nevus sebaceus of Jadassohn. Arch Dermatol 1965;91:574–88.
20. Domingo J, Helwig EB. Malignant neoplasms associated with nevus sebaceus of Jadassohn. J Am Acad Dermatol 1979;1(6):545–56.
21. Chun K, Vazquez M, Sanchez JL. Nevus sebaceus: clinical outcome and considerations for prophylactic excision. Int J Dermatol 1995;34(8):538–41.
22. Serrano R, Lopez-Rios F, Rodriguez-Peralto JL. Tumors arising in nevus sebaceus. J Am Acad Dermatol 2001;45(5):792 [author reply: 794].
23. Santibanez-Gallerani A, Marshall D, Duarte AM, et al. Should nevus sebaceus of Jadassohn in children be excised? A study of 757 cases, and literature review. J Craniofac Surg 2003;14(5):658–60.
24. Duncan A, Wilson N, Leonard N. Squamous cell carcinoma developing in a naevus sebaceous of Jadassohn. Am J Dermatopathol 2008;30(3):269–70.
25. Kazakov DV, Calonje E, Zelger B, et al. Sebaceous carcinoma arising in nevus sebaceus of Jadassohn: a clinicopathological study of five cases. Am J Dermatopathol 2007;29(3):242–8.
26. Misago N, Kodera H, Narisawa Y. Sebaceous carcinoma, trichoblastoma, and sebaceoma with features of trichoblastoma in nevus sebaceus. Am J Dermatopathol 2001;23(5):456–62.

27. Miller CJ, Ioffreda MD, Billingsley EM. Sebaceous carcinoma, basal cell carcinoma, trichoadenoma, trichoblastoma, and syringocystadenoma papilliferum arising within a nevus sebaceus. Dermatol Surg 2004;30(12 Pt 2):1546–9.
28. Tarkhan II, Domingo J. Metastasizing eccrine porocarcinoma developing in a sebaceous nevus of Jadassohn. Report of a case. Arch Dermatol 1985; 121(3):413–5.
29. Kantrow SM, Ivan D, Williams MD, et al. Metastasizing adenocarcinoma and multiple neoplastic proliferations arising in a nevus sebaceus. Am J Dermatopathol 2007;29(5):462–6.
30. Manonukul J, Omeapinyan P, Vongjirad A. Mucoepidermoid (adenosquamous) carcinoma, trichoblastoma, trichilemmoma, sebaceous adenoma, tumor of follicular infundibulum and syringocystadenoma papilliferum arising within 2 persistent lesions of nevus sebaceous: report of a case. Am J Dermatopathol 2009;31:658–63.
31. Barkham MC, White N, Brundler MA, et al. Should naevus sebaceus be excised prophylactically? A clinical audit. J Plast Reconstr Aesthet Surg 2007;60(11):1269–70.
32. Altaykan A, Ersoy-Evans S, Erkin G, et al. Basal cell carcinoma arising in nevus sebaceous during childhood. Pediatr Dermatol 2008;25(6):616–9.
33. Belhadjali H, Moussa A, Yahia S, et al. Simultaneous occurrence of two squamous cell carcinomas within a nevus sebaceous of Jadassohn in an 11-year-old girl. Pediatr Dermatol 2009;26(2):236–7.
34. Hidvegi NC, Kangesu L, Wolfe KQ. Squamous cell carcinoma complicating naevus sebaceous of Jadassohn in a child. Br J Plast Surg 2003;56(1):50–2.
35. Hughes SM, Wilkerson AE, Winfield HL, et al. Familial nevus sebaceus in dizygotic male twins. J Am Acad Dermatol 2006;54(Suppl 2):S47–8.
36. Laino L, Steensel MA, Innocenzi D, et al. Familial occurrence of nevus sebaceus of Jadassohn: another case of paradominant inheritance? Eur J Dermatol 2001; 11(2):97–8.
37. Sahl WJ Jr. Familial nevus sebaceus of Jadassohn: occurrence in three generations. J Am Acad Dermatol 1990;22(5 Pt 1):853–4.
38. Monk BE, Vollum DI. Familial naevus sebaceus. J R Soc Med 1982;75(8):660–1.
39. Fearfield LA, Bunker CB. Familial naevus sebaceous of Jadassohn. Br J Dermatol 1998;139(6):1119–20.
40. Happle R, Konig A. Familial naevus sebaceus may be explained by paradominant transmission. Br J Dermatol 1999;141(2):377.
41. Carlson JA, Cribier B, Nuovo G, et al. Epidermodysplasia verruciformis-associated and genital-mucosal high-risk human papillomavirus DNA are prevalent in nevus sebaceus of Jadassohn. J Am Acad Dermatol 2008;59(2):279–94.
42. Xin H, Matt D, Qin JZ, et al. The sebaceous nevus: a nevus with deletions of the PTCH gene. Cancer Res 1999;59(8):1834–6.
43. Mckee PH, Calonje E, Granter SR. Nevus sebaceus. In: Mckee PH, Calonje E, Granter SR, editors. London: Elsevier Mosby; 2005. p. 1568.
44. Eisen DB, Michael DJ. Sebaceous lesions and their associated syndromes: part I. J Am Acad Dermatol 2009;61(4):549–60 [quiz: 561–2].
45. Orchard DC, Weston WL, Morelli JG. Tumors arising in nevus sebaceus. J Am Acad Dermatol 2001;45(5):793–4 [author reply: 794].
46. Ashinoff R. Linear nevus sebaceus of Jadassohn treated with the carbon dioxide laser. Pediatr Dermatol 1993;10(2):189–91.
47. Dierickx CC, Goldenhersh M, Dwyer P, et al. Photodynamic therapy for nevus sebaceus with topical delta-aminolevulinic acid. Arch Dermatol 1999;135(6): 637–40.

48. Cestari TF, Rubim M, Valentini BC. Nevus comedonicus: case report and brief review of the literature. Pediatr Dermatol 1991;8(4):300–5.
49. Kirtak N, Inaloz HS, Karakok M, et al. Extensive inflammatory nevus comedonicus involving half of the body. Int J Dermatol 2004;43(6):434–6.
50. Lefkowitz A, Schwartz RA, Lambert WC. Nevus comedonicus. Dermatology 1999;199(3):204–7.
51. Wakahara M, Kiyohara T, Kumakiri M, et al. Bilateral nevus comedonicus: efficacy of topical tacalcitol ointment. Acta Derm Venereol 2003;83(1):51.
52. Deliduka SB, Kwong PC. Treatment of nevus comedonicus with topical tazarotene and calcipotriene. J Drugs Dermatol 2004;3(6):674–6.
53. Vasiloudes PE, Morelli JG, Weston WL. Inflammatory nevus comedonicus in children. J Am Acad Dermatol 1998;38(5 Pt 2):834–6.
54. Alpsoy E, Durusoy C, Ozbilim G, et al. Nevus comedonicus syndrome: a case associated with multiple basal cell carcinomas and a rudimentary toe. Int J Dermatol 2005;44(6):499–501.
55. Walling HW, Swick BL. Squamous cell carcinoma arising in nevus comedonicus. Dermatol Surg 2009;35(1):144–6.
56. Wood MG, Thew MA. Nevus comedonicus. A case with palmar involvement and review of the literature. Arch Dermatol 1968;98(2):111–6.
57. Barsky S, Doyle JA, Winkelmann RK. Nevus comedonicus with epidermolytic hyperkeratosis. A report of four cases. Arch Dermatol 1981;117(2):86–8.
58. Munro CS, Wilkie AO. Epidermal mosaicism producing localised acne: somatic mutation in FGFR2. Lancet 1998;352(9129):704–5.
59. Kurokawa I, Nakai Y, Nishimura K, et al. Cytokeratin and filaggrin expression in nevus comedonicus. J Cutan Pathol 2007;34(4):338–41.
60. Morillo V, Manrique P, De Miguel E, et al. Nevus comedonicus with epidermolytic hyperkeratosis. Eur J Dermatol 2007;17(2):176–7.
61. Lookingbill DP, Ladda RL, Cohen C. Generalized epidermolytic hyperkeratosis in the child of a parent with nevus comedonicus. Arch Dermatol 1984;120(2):223–6.
62. Milton GP, DiGiovanna JJ, Peck GL. Treatment of nevus comedonicus with ammonium lactate lotion. J Am Acad Dermatol 1989;20(2 Pt 2):324–8.
63. Beck MH, Dave VK. Extensive nevus comedonicus. Arch Dermatol 1980;116(9):1048–50.
64. Caers SJ, Van der Geer S, Beverdam EG, et al. Successful treatment of nevus comedonicus with the use of the erbium YAG laser. J Eur Acad Dermatol Venereol 2008;22(3):375–7.
65. Inoue Y, Miyamoto Y, Ono T. Two cases of nevus comedonicus: successful treatment of keratin plugs with a pore strip. J Am Acad Dermatol 2000;43(5 Pt 2):927–9.
66. Tymen R, Forestier JF, Boutet B, et al. Late Becker's nevus. One hundred cases (author's translation). Ann Dermatol Venereol 1981;108(1):41–6.
67. Ballone E, Fazii P, Lappa G, et al. Prevalence of Becker's nevi in a population of young men in central Italy. J Am Acad Dermatol 2003;48(5):795.
68. Ingordo V, Gentile C, Iannazzone SS, et al. The 'EpiEnlist' project: a dermo-epidemiologic study on a representative sample of young Italian males. Prevalence of selected pigmentary lesions. J Eur Acad Dermatol Venereol 2007;21(8):1091–6.
69. Hsu S, Chen JY, Subrt P. Becker's melanosis in a woman. J Am Acad Dermatol 2001;45(Suppl 6):S195–6.
70. Happle R. Epidermal nevus syndromes. Semin Dermatol 1995;14(2):111–21.

71. Sood A, D'Souza P, Verma KK. Becker's naevus occurring at birth and in early childhood. Acta Derm Venereol 1998;78(4):311.
72. Book SE, Glass AT, Laude TA. Congenital Becker's nevus with a familial association. Pediatr Dermatol 1997;14(5):373-5.
73. Kilic A, Kaya I, Gul U, et al. Becker nevus on face with asymmetrical growth of beard hair. J Eur Acad Dermatol Venereol 2008;22(2):246-7.
74. de Almeida HL Jr, Happle R. Two cases of cephalic Becker nevus with asymmetrical growth of beard or scalp hair. Dermatology 2003;207(3):337-8.
75. Alhusayen R, Kanigsberg N, Jackson R. Becker nevus on the lower limb: case report and review of the literature. J Cutan Med Surg 2008;12(1):31-4.
76. Khaitan BK, Manchanda Y, Mittal R, et al. Multiple Becker's naevi: a rare presentation. Acta Derm Venereol 2001;81(5):374-5.
77. Khatami A, Seradj MH, Gorouhi F, et al. Giant bilateral Becker nevus: a rare presentation. Pediatr Dermatol 2008;25(1):47-51.
78. Grim KD, Wasko CA. Symmetrical bilateral Becker melanosis: a rare presentation. Dermatol Online J 2009;15(12):1.
79. Panizzon RG. Familial Becker's nevus. Int J Dermatol 1990;29(2):158.
80. Happle R. What is paradominant inheritance? J Med Genet 2009;46(9):648.
81. Urbani CE. Paradominant inheritance, supernumerary nipples and Becker's nevus: once again! Eur J Dermatol 2001;11(6):597.
82. Person JR, Longcope C. Becker's nevus: an androgen-mediated hyperplasia with increased androgen receptors. J Am Acad Dermatol 1984;10(2 Pt 1): 235-8.
83. Grande Sarpa H, Harris R, Hansen CD, et al. Androgen receptor expression patterns in Becker's nevi: an immunohistochemical study. J Am Acad Dermatol 2008;59(5):834-8.
84. Nirde P, Dereure O, Belon C, et al. The association of Becker nevus with hypersensitivity to androgens. Arch Dermatol 1999;135(2):212-4.
85. Mckee PH, Calonje E, Granter SR. Becker's nevus. In: Mckee PH, Calonje E, Granter SR, editors. London: Elsevier Mosby; 2005. p. 1249.
86. Ingordo V, Iannazzone SS, Cusano F, et al. Dermoscopic features of congenital melanocytic nevus and Becker nevus in an adult male population: an analysis with a 10-fold magnification. Dermatology 2006;212(4):354-60.
87. Fehr B, Panizzon RG, Schnyder UW. Becker's nevus and malignant melanoma. Dermatologica 1991;182(2):77-80.
88. Honda M, Suzuki T, Kudoh K, et al. Bowen's disease developing within a Becker's melanosis (Becker's naevus). Br J Dermatol 1997;137(4):659-61.
89. Patrizi A, Medri M, Neri I, et al. Becker naevus associated with basal cell carcinoma, melanocytic naevus and smooth-muscle hamartoma. J Eur Acad Dermatol Venereol 2007;21(1):130-2.
90. Trelles MA, Allones I, Moreno-Arias GA, et al. Becker's naevus: a comparative study between erbium: YAG and Q-switched neodymium:YAG; clinical and histopathological findings. Br J Dermatol 2005;152(2):308-13.
91. Choi JE, Kim JW, Seo SH, et al. Treatment of Becker's nevi with a long-pulse alexandrite laser. Dermatol Surg 2009;35(7):1105-8.
92. Glaich AS, Goldberg LH, Dai T, et al. Fractional resurfacing: a new therapeutic modality for Becker's nevus. Arch Dermatol 2007;143(12):1488-90.
93. Morag C, Metzker A. Inflammatory linear verrucous epidermal nevus: report of seven new cases and review of the literature. Pediatr Dermatol 1985;3:15-8.
94. Lee SH, Rogers M. Inflammatory linear verrucous epidermal naevi: a review of 25 cases. Aust J Dermatol 2001;42:252-6.

95. Lee BJ, Mancini AJ, Renucci J, et al. Full-thickness surgical excision for the treatment of inflammatory linear verrucous epidermal nevus. Ann Plast Surg 2001;47:285–92.
96. Cambiaghi S, Gianotti R, Caputo R. Widespread porokeratotic eccrine ostial and dermal duct nevus along Blaschko lines. Pediatr Dermatol 2007;24(2):162–7.
97. Goddard DS, Rogers M, Frieden IJ, et al. Widespread porokeratotic adnexal ostial nevus: clinical features and proposal of a new name unifying porokeratotic eccrine ostial and dermal duct nevus and porokeratotic eccrine and hair follicle nevus. J Am Acad Dermatol 2009;61(6):1060. e1–14.
98. Jamora MJ, Celis MA. Generalized porokeratotic eccrine ostial and dermal duct nevus associated with deafness. J Am Acad Dermatol 2008;59(2 Suppl 1):S43–5.
99. Valks R, Abajo P, Fraga J, et al. Porokeratotic eccrine ostial and dermal duct nevus of late onset: more frequent than previously suggested? Dermatology 1996;193(2):138–40.
100. Birol A, Erkek E, Bozdoethan O, et al. A case of porokeratotic eccrine ostial and dermal duct naevus of late onset. J Eur Acad Dermatol Venereol 2004;18(5):619–21.
101. van de Kerkhof PC, Steijlen PM, Happle R. Co-occurrence of linear psoriasis and porokeratotic eccrine ostial and dermal duct naevus. Acta Derm Venereol 1993;73(4):311–2.
102. Yu HJ, Ko JY, Kwon HM, et al. Linear psoriasis with porokeratotic eccrine ostial and dermal duct nevus. J Am Acad Dermatol 2004;50(Suppl 5):S81–3.
103. Nassiri N, Hansen J. Diffuse squamous cell carcinoma in porokeratotic eccrine ostial and dermal duct nevus. Plast Reconstr Surg 2009;123(2):87e–8e.
104. Coras B, Vogt T, Roesch A, et al. Bowen's disease on porokeratotic eccrine ostial and dermal duct nevus. Dermatol Surg 2007;33(4):496–9.
105. Solis J, Sau P, James WD. Puzzling palmar and plantar papules. Porokeratotic eccrine ostial and dermal duct nevus. Arch Dermatol 1991;127(8):1220–1, 1223–4.
106. Sassmannshausen J, Bogomilsky J, Chaffins M. Porokeratotic eccrine ostial and dermal duct nevus: a case report and review of the literature. J Am Acad Dermatol 2000;43(2 Pt 2):364–7.
107. Masferrer E, Vicente A, Bassas-Vila J, et al. Porokeratotic eccrine ostial and dermal duct naevus: report of 10 cases. J Eur Acad Dermatol Venereol 2010;24(7):847–51.
108. Wang NS, Meola T, Orlow SJ, et al. Porokeratotic eccrine ostial and dermal duct nevus: a report of 2 cases and review of the literature. Am J Dermatopathol 2009;31(6):582–6.
109. Leung CS, Tang WY, Lam WY, et al. Porokeratotic eccrine ostial and dermal duct naevus with dermatomal trunk involvement: literature review and report on the efficacy of laser treatment. Br J Dermatol 1998;138(4):684–8.
110. Del Pozo J, Martinez W, Verea MM, et al. Porokeratotic eccrine ostial and dermal duct naevus: treatment with carbon dioxide laser. Br J Dermatol 1999;141(6):1144–5.
111. Mazuecos J, Ortega M, Rios JJ, et al. Long-term involution of unilateral porokeratotic eccrine ostial and dermal duct naevus. Acta Derm Venereol 2003;83(2):147–9.
112. Aloi FG, Pippione M. Porokeratotic eccrine ostial and dermal duct nevus. Arch Dermatol 1986;122(8):892–5.
113. Ivker R, Resnick SD, Skidmore RA. Hypophosphatemic vitamin D-resistant rickets, precocious puberty, and the epidermal nevus syndrome. Arch Dermatol 1997;133:1557–61.

114. Biesecker L. The challenges of Proteus syndrome: diagnosis and management. Eur J Hum Genet 2006;14(11):1151–7.
115. Cohen MM Jr. Proteus syndrome: an update. Am J Med Genet C Semin Med Genet 2005;137C(1):38–52.
116. Biesecker LG, Happle R, Mulliken JB, et al. Proteus syndrome: diagnostic criteria, differential diagnosis, and patient evaluation. Am J Med Genet 1999; 84(5):389–95.
117. Turner JT, Cohen MM Jr, Biesecker LG. Reassessment of the Proteus syndrome literature: application of diagnostic criteria to published cases. Am J Med Genet A 2004;130(2):111–22.
118. Biesecker LG, Peters KF, Darling TN, et al. Clinical differentiation between Proteus syndrome and hemihyperplasia: description of a distinct form of hemihyperplasia. Am J Med Genet 1998;79(4):311–8.
119. Nguyen D, Turner JT, Olsen C, et al. Cutaneous manifestations of Proteus syndrome: correlations with general clinical severity. Arch Dermatol 2004; 140(8):947–53.
120. Happle R. Lethal genes surviving by mosaicism: a possible explanation for sporadic birth defects involving the skin. J Am Acad Dermatol 1987;16(4): 899–906.
121. Cohen MM Jr. Proteus syndrome: clinical evidence for somatic mosaicism and selective review. Am J Med Genet 1993;47(5):645–52.
122. Liaw D, Marsh DJ, Li J, et al. Germline mutations of the PTEN gene in Cowden disease, an inherited breast and thyroid cancer syndrome. Nat Genet 1997; 16(1):64–7.
123. Nelen MR, van Staveren WC, Peeters EA, et al. Germline mutations in the PTEN/MMAC1 gene in patients with Cowden disease. Hum Mol Genet 1997;6(8): 1383–7.
124. Arch EM, Goodman BK, Van Wesep RA, et al. Deletion of PTEN in a patient with Bannayan-Riley-Ruvalcaba syndrome suggests allelism with Cowden disease. Am J Med Genet 1997;71(4):489–93.
125. Marsh DJ, Coulon V, Lunetta KL, et al. Mutation spectrum and genotype-phenotype analyses in Cowden disease and Bannayan-Zonana syndrome, two hamartoma syndromes with germline PTEN mutation. Hum Mol Genet 1998;7(3): 507–15.
126. Zhou X, Hampel H, Thiele H, et al. Association of germline mutation in the PTEN tumour suppressor gene and Proteus and Proteus-like syndromes. Lancet 2001; 358(9277):210–1.
127. Smith JM, Kirk EP, Theodosopoulos G, et al. Germline mutation of the tumour suppressor PTEN in Proteus syndrome. J Med Genet 2002;39(12):937–40.
128. Loffeld A, McLellan NJ, Cole T, et al. Epidermal naevus in Proteus syndrome showing loss of heterozygosity for an inherited PTEN mutation. Br J Dermatol 2006;154(6):1194–8.
129. Biesecker LG, Rosenberg MJ, Vacha S, et al. PTEN mutations and Proteus syndrome. Lancet 2001;358(9298):2079–80.
130. Cohen MM Jr, Turner JT, Biesecker LG. Proteus syndrome: misdiagnosis with PTEN mutations. Am J Med Genet A 2003;122(4):323–4.
131. Barker K, Martinez A, Wang R, et al. PTEN mutations are uncommon in Proteus syndrome. J Med Genet 2001;38(7):480–1.
132. Thiffault I, Schwartz CE, Der Kaloustian V, et al. Mutation analysis of the tumor suppressor PTEN and the glypican 3 (GPC3) gene in patients diagnosed with Proteus syndrome. Am J Med Genet A 2004;130(2):123–7.

133. Happle R. Type 2 segmental Cowden disease vs. Proteus syndrome. Br J Dermatol 2007;156(5):1089–90.
134. Happle R. Linear Cowden nevus: a new distinct epidermal nevus. Eur J Dermatol 2007;17(2):133–6.
135. Slavotinek AM, Vacha SJ, Peters KF, et al. Sudden death caused by pulmonary thromboembolism in Proteus syndrome. Clin Genet 2000;58(5):386–9.
136. Cohen MM Jr. Causes of premature death in Proteus syndrome. Am J Med Genet 2001;101(1):1–3.
137. Turner J, Biesecker B, Leib J, et al. Parenting children with Proteus syndrome: experiences with, and adaptation to, courtesy stigma. Am J Med Genet A 2007;143(18):2089–97.
138. Biesecker LG. The multifaceted challenges of Proteus syndrome. JAMA 2001;285(17):2240–3.
139. Caux F, Plauchu H, Chibon F, et al. Segmental overgrowth, lipomatosis, arteriovenous malformation and epidermal nevus (SOLAMEN) syndrome is related to mosaic PTEN nullizygosity. Eur J Hum Genet 2007;15(7):767–73.
140. Sapp JC, Turner JT, van de Kamp JM, et al. Newly delineated syndrome of congenital lipomatous overgrowth, vascular malformations, and epidermal nevi (CLOVE syndrome) in seven patients. Am J Med Genet A 2007;143(24):2944–58.
141. Gucev ZS, Tasic V, Jancevska A, et al. Congenital lipomatous overgrowth, vascular malformations, and epidermal nevi (CLOVE) syndrome: CNS malformations and seizures may be a component of this disorder. Am J Med Genet A 2008;146(20):2688–90.
142. McCall S, Ramzy MI, Cure JK, et al. Encephalocraniocutaneous lipomatosis and the Proteus syndrome: distinct entities with overlapping manifestations. Am J Med Genet 1992;43(4):662–8.
143. Alomari AI. Characterization of a distinct syndrome that associates complex truncal overgrowth, vascular, and acral anomalies: a descriptive study of 18 cases of CLOVES syndrome. Clin Dysmorphol 2009;18(1):1–7.
144. Alomari AI. CLOVE(S) syndrome: expanding the acronym. Am J Med Genet A 2009;149(2):294; author reply 295.
145. Fernandez-Pineda I, Fajardo M, Chaudry G, et al. Perinatal clinical and imaging features of CLOVES syndrome. Pediatr Radiol 2010;40:1436–9.
146. van de Warrenburg BP, van Gulik S, Renier WO, et al. The linear naevus sebaceus syndrome. Clin Neurol Neurosurg 1998;100(2):126–32.
147. Davies D, Rogers M. Review of neurological manifestations in 196 patients with sebaceous naevi. Australas J Dermatol 2002;43(1):20–3.
148. Menascu S, Donner EJ. Linear nevus sebaceous syndrome: case reports and review of the literature. Pediatr Neurol 2008;38(3):207–10.
149. Vidaurri-de la Cruz H, Tamayo-Sanchez L, Duran-McKinster C, et al. Epidermal nevus syndromes: clinical findings in 35 patients. Pediatr Dermatol 2004;21(4):432–9.
150. Zutt M, Strutz F, Happle R, et al. Schimmelpenning-Feuerstein-Mims syndrome with hypophosphatemic rickets. Dermatology 2003;207(1):72–6.
151. Warnke PH, Schimmelpenning GW, Happle R, et al. Intraoral lesions associated with sebaceous nevus syndrome. J Cutan Pathol 2006;33(2):175–80.
152. Happle R, Konig A. Didymosis aplasticosebacea: coexistence of aplasia cutis congenita and nevus sebaceus may be explained as a twin spot phenomenon. Dermatology 2001;202(3):246–8.

153. Demerdjieva Z, Kavaklieva S, Tsankov N. Epidermal nevus syndrome and didymosis aplasticosebacea. Pediatr Dermatol 2007;24(5):514-6.
154. Lam J, Dohil MA, Eichenfield LF, et al. SCALP syndrome: sebaceous nevus syndrome, CNS malformations, aplasia cutis congenita, limbal dermoid, and pigmented nevus (giant) congenital melanocytic nevus with neurocutaneous melanosis: a distinct syndromic entity. J Am Acad Dermatol 2008;58(5):884-8.
155. Eisen DB, Michael DJ. Sebaceous lesions and their associated syndromes: part II. J Am Acad Dermatol 2009;61(4):563-78; quiz 579-80.
156. Happle R, Hoffmann R, Restano L, et al. Phacomatosis pigmentokeratotica: a melanocytic-epidermal twin nevus syndrome. Am J Med Genet 1996;65(4):363-5.
157. Torrelo A, Zambrano A. What syndrome is this. Phakomatosis pigmentokeratotica (Happle). Pediatr Dermatol 1998;15(4):321-3.
158. Gruson LM, Orlow SJ, Schaffer JV. Phacomatosis pigmentokeratotica associated with hemihypertrophy and a rhabdomyosarcoma of the abdominal wall. J Am Acad Dermatol 2006;55(Suppl 2):S16-20.
159. Polat M, Yalcin B, Ustun H, et al. Phacomatosis pigmentokeratotica without extracutaneous abnormalities. Eur J Dermatol 2008;18(3):363-4.
160. Wollenberg A, Butnaru C, Oppel T. Phacomatosis pigmentokeratotica (Happle) in a 23-year-old man. Acta Derm Venereol 2002;82(1):55-7.
161. Kinoshita K, Shinkai H, Utani A. Phacomatosis pigmentokeratotica without extracutaneous abnormalities. Dermatology 2003;207(4):415-6.
162. Tadini G, Restano L, Gonzales-Perez R, et al. Phacomatosis pigmentokeratotica: report of new cases and further delineation of the syndrome. Arch Dermatol 1998;134(3):333-7.
163. Martinez-Menchon T, Mahiques Santos L, Vilata Corell JJ, et al. Phacomatosis pigmentokeratotica: a 20-year follow-up with malignant degeneration of both nevus components. Pediatr Dermatol 2005;22(1):44-7.
164. Bouthors J, Vantyghem MC, Manouvrier-Hanu S, et al. Phacomatosis pigmentokeratotica associated with hypophosphataemic rickets, pheochromocytoma and multiple basal cell carcinomas. Br J Dermatol 2006;155(1):225-6.
165. Okada E, Tamura A, Ishikawa O. Phacomatosis pigmentokeratotica complicated with juvenile onset hypertension. Acta Derm Venereol 2004;84(5):397-8.
166. Boente MC, Pizzi de Parra N, Larralde de Luna M, et al. Phacomatosis pigmentokeratotica: another epidermal nevus syndrome and a distinctive type of twin spotting. Eur J Dermatol 2000;10(3):190-4.
167. Patrizi A, Neri I, Fiorentini C, et al. Nevus comedonicus syndrome: a new pediatric case. Pediatr Dermatol 1998;15(4):304-6.
168. Seo YJ, Piao YJ, Suhr KB, et al. A case of nevus comedonicus syndrome associated with neurologic and skeletal abnormalities. Int J Dermatol 2001;40(10):648-50.
169. Guldbakke KK, Khachemoune A, Deng A, et al. Naevus comedonicus: a spectrum of body involvement. Clin Exp Dermatol 2007;32(5):488-92.
170. Filosa G, Bugatti L, Ciattaglia G, et al. Naevus comedonicus as dermatologic hallmark of occult spinal dysraphism. Acta Derm Venereol 1997;77(3):243.
171. Happle R, Koopman RJ. Becker nevus syndrome. Am J Med Genet 1997;68(3):357-61.
172. Danarti R, Konig A, Salhi A, et al. Becker's nevus syndrome revisited. J Am Acad Dermatol 2004;51(6):965-9.
173. Welsch MJ, Stein SL. A syndrome of hemimaxillary enlargement, asymmetry of the face, tooth abnormalities, and skin findings (HATS). Pediatr Dermatol 2004;21(4):448-51.

174. Urbani CE, Betti R. Supernumerary nipple in association with Becker nevus vs. Becker nevus syndrome: a semantic problem only. Am J Med Genet 1998;77(1): 76–7.
175. Urbani CE, Betti R. Supernumerary nipples occurring together with Becker's naevus: an association involving one common paradominant trait? Hum Genet 1997;100(3–4):388–90.
176. Cheng J, Syder AJ, Yu QC, et al. The genetic basis of epidermolytic hyperkeratosis: a disorder of differentiation-specific epidermal keratin genes. Cell 1992; 70(5):811–9.
177. Syder AJ, Yu QC, Paller AS, et al. Genetic mutations in the K1 and K10 genes of patients with epidermolytic hyperkeratosis. Correlation between location and disease severity. J Clin Invest 1994;93(4):1533–42.
178. McLean WH, Morley SM, Lane EB, et al. Ichthyosis bullosa of Siemens-A disease involving keratin 2e. J Invest Dermatol 1994;103(3):277–81.
179. Rothnagel JA, Traupe H, Wojcik S, et al. Mutations in the rod domain of keratin 2e in patients with ichthyosis bullosa of Siemens. Nat Genet 1994;7(4):485–90.
180. Happle R. Ptychotropism as a cutaneous feature of the CHILD syndrome. J Am Acad Dermatol 1990;23(4 Pt 1):763–6.
181. Konig A, Happle R, Bornholdt D, et al. Mutations in the NSDHL gene, encoding a 3beta-hydroxysteroid dehydrogenase, cause CHILD syndrome. Am J Med Genet 2000;90(4):339–46.
182. Happle R, Effendy I, Megahed M, et al. CHILD syndrome in a boy. Am J Med Genet 1996;62(2):192–4.

Index

Note: Page numbers of article titles are in **boldface** type.

A

Acanthosis, in nevus sebaceous, 1180
Acoustic schwannomas, 1143
Airway, hemangiomas of, 1075–1076
Aminocaproic acid, for Kasabach-Merritt phenomenon, 1087
Anemia
   Fanconi, 1137
   in Kasabach-Merritt phenomenon, 1085–1086
Angel's kiss, 1093
Angiogenesis, in infantile hemangioma, 1070
Angiomas
   tufted, 1085–1088
   venous or cavernous. *See* Venous malformations.
Antiplatelet agents, for Kasabach-Merritt phenomenon, 1087
Aortic anomalies, in PHACE syndrome, 1076–1078
Aplasia cutis congenita, in nevus sebaceous syndrome, 1187
Arterial abnormalities, in PHACE syndrome, 1076–1078
Arteriovenous malformations
   capillary malformations with, 1105, 1112, 1114–1115
   clinical characteristics of, 1104
   diagnosis of, 1105
   syndromes associated with, 1095, 1104–1105, 1113
   treatment of, 1105
Ataxia-telangiectasia, 1136

B

Bannayan-Riley-Ruvalcaba syndrome
   café-au-lait macules in, 1136
   vascular malformations in, 1095
Barrier creams, for hemangiomas, 1078–1079
Bathing trunk nevi. *See* Congenital melanocytic nevi.
Bean syndrome (blue rubber bleb nevus syndrome), 1094, 1099, 1113
Becaplermin gel, for hemangiomas, 1078–1079
Becker nevi, 1133–1134, 1181–1183, 1188
Beckwith-Wiedemann syndrome, 1094
Benign neonatal hemangiomatosis, 1075
Birthmarks
   café-au-lait macules, 1124, **1131–1153**
   hemangiomas, **1069–1083,** 1159
   in Kasabach-Merritt phenomenon, **1085–1089**

Pediatr Clin N Am 57 (2010) 1199–1210
doi:10.1016/S0031-3955(10)00140-9
0031-3955/10/$ – see front matter © 2010 Elsevier Inc. All rights reserved.

pediatric.theclinics.com